CLINICIAN'S GUIDE TO PARTIAL HOSPITALIZATION AND INTENSIVE OUTPATIENT PRACTICE

David Houvenagle, PhD, LCSW, earned his BA from Iowa State University, Ames, Iowa; his Master's of Divinity from Bethel University, St. Paul, Minnesota; and his Master's of Social Work from the Southern Baptist Theological Seminary, Louisville, Kentucky. He earned his PhD in urban and public affairs from the University of Louisville, Louisville, Kentucky, with an emphasis on policy and administration. His previous published work is *Local Healthcare Politics: Louisville's Growth Machine 1947–2007.*

Dr. Houvenagle has been a social worker for over 20 years. He has been a clinician in the psychiatric setting for over 18 years and has been working in the partial hospitalization and intensive outpatient program settings for more than 12 years.

CLINICIAN'S GUIDE TO PARTIAL HOSPITALIZATION AND INTENSIVE OUTPATIENT PRACTICE

David Houvenagle, PhD, LCSW

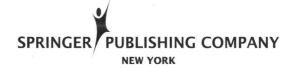

SPRINGER PUBLISHING COMPANY
NEW YORK

Springer Publishing Company, LLC
11 West 42nd Street
New York, NY 10036
www.springerpub.com

Acquisitions Editor: Stephanie Drew
Composition: Exeter Premedia Services Private Ltd.

ISBN: 978-0-8261-2882-9
e-book ISBN: 978-0-8261-2883-6
Sample Handouts ISBN: 978-0-8261-2879-9

Sample Handouts are available from *www.springerpub.com/houvenagle*

15 16 17 18 19 / 5 4 3 2 1

The author and the publisher of this Work have made every effort to use sources believed to be reliable to provide information that is accurate and compatible with the standards generally accepted at the time of publication. The author and publisher shall not be liable for any special, consequential, or exemplary damages resulting, in whole or in part, from the readers' use of, or reliance on, the information contained in this book. The publisher has no responsibility for the persistence or accuracy of URLs for external or third-party Internet websites referred to in this publication and does not guarantee that any content on such websites is, or will remain, accurate or appropriate.

Library of Congress Cataloging-in-Publication Data
Houvenagle, David, author.
Clinician's guide to partial hospitalization and intensive outpatient practice / David Houvenagle.
  p. ; cm.
Includes bibliographical references and index.
  ISBN 978-0-8261-2882-9—ISBN 978-0-8261-2883-6 (e-book)
  I. Title.
  [DNLM: 1. Ambulatory Care. 2. Ambulatory Care Facilities—organization & administration.
  3. Continuity of Patient Care. 4. Day Care. WB 101]
  RA974
  362.12—dc23
                                                                        2015002716

Special discounts on bulk quantities of our books are available to corporations, professional associations, pharmaceutical companies, health care organizations, and other qualifying groups. If you are interested in a custom book, including chapters from more than one of our titles, we can provide that service as well.

For details, please contact:
Special Sales Department, Springer Publishing Company, LLC
11 West 42nd Street, 15th Floor, New York, NY 10036-8002
Phone: 877-687-7476 or 212-431-4370; Fax: 212-941-7842
E-mail: sales@springerpub.com

Printed in the United States of America by Gasch Printing.

To Tim Bowman, LCSW

As iron sharpens iron, so one man sharpens another.
—Proverbs 27:17 (New International Version)

CONTENTS

PREFACE

This book emerged as a result of the supervision of a supervisee toward the Licensed Clinical Social Worker credential. Although much of this material could be used in other clinical supervision and field education contexts, this book seeks to guide a master's-level clinician with rudimentary, clinical knowledge of professional practice and development within the partial hospitalization program and intensive outpatient program (PHP/IOP) settings.

There is a dearth of material on evidence-based practice in this clinical setting. Therefore, this book is based on the writer's experience of more than 12 years of clinical work in five different PHP/IOP cohorts and further graduate work in urban and public affairs at the University of Louisville, Louisville, Kentucky. The graduate work provided some opportunity to think outside of the box about the conduct of clinical work through exposure to other theoretical concepts.

This book borrows from the school of urban political economy and a preexisting political science theory called the *ecology of games* to create a consistent and orderly conception of the salient practice areas and issues in the PHP/IOP setting. Although the term *game* can have an inflammatory connotation, it merely refers to a set of strategies. Each chapter is an exploration of the puzzle found in each practice area or cohort and the game or set of strategies used to address the puzzle. Because each puzzle is different, the set of practice strategies varies as to the level of abstraction and precision.

Sample handouts that can be used in psychoeducational sessions are available for download from Springer Publishing Company's website: www.springerpub.com/houvenagle.

Acknowledgments

Many thanks are due to the following people who have assisted in writing this book. I leaned on their feedback, guidance, and support.

Jim Brock, PsyD, has been an early and continued supporter of this project since long before I got the Springer Publishing Company contract. He reviewed most of the chapters for content, style, and grammar and pulled no punches when I needed to hear difficult criticism, for which I am most thankful. He is one of the most gracious people on the planet.

Anne Faulls was once again generous enough to edit the grammar in this book after editing my PhD dissertation from the University of Louisville. She is a very kind, Christian woman, and I am thankful for her generosity.

The following professionals read different chapters and gave valuable feedback: Bruce Conn, LMFT; Dianne Doyle, LCSW; Ruth Gabehart, RN, MSW; Kristina Knebel-Hutchinson, MA; Ann Hutton, RN; Eric Marcum, RN; Gretchen Rinehart, LCSW, CADC; John E. Schmanski II, MEd; Brenda Short, LCSW; Michael Taylor, LMFT; and Julian Pace, MHA. I thank them for their time and thoughts.

Thanks must be given to the love of my life, Leslie, and our children, Aimee and Stephen, for their forbearance. This project monopolized our lives for several months.

CHAPTER ONE

INTRODUCTION

*T*he partial hospitalization program (PHP) and intensive outpatient program (IOP) have evolved as significant services in the continuum of care for mental health treatment. They have proven to be effective, efficient, and relatively inexpensive services. It is likely that these settings will continue to evolve in terms of both diversity and size as new treatment populations are identified as appropriate for this level of care. Despite the advantages, these intense treatment settings are demanding and often difficult work environments. Little has been written about them in terms of practice. The focus of this book is on understanding what will create successful, sound, and sustainable program delivery in these settings.

This chapter offers an introductory overview of these programs. It reviews the theoretical nature of the PHP/IOP levels of care and the recurring theoretical themes and paradigms in this book, which include the concepts of *games, continuity,* and *reasonable expectations*. It closes with an overview of the book.

PHP AND IOP WITHIN THE CONTINUUM OF SERVICES

The psychiatric services system can be described on a continuum of severity (Figure 1.1). At the severe end is inpatient care. The least severe end is the self-help group. The most severe case is a patient forcibly committed to inpatient care by the order of a judge or magistrate for being a danger to self or others. The least severe case would be a well-functioning person independently going to a support group out of a strong personal desire and not suffering any significant consequences when ceasing attendance.

Otherwise, determining the appropriate level of care for a patient has to do with the mix of the patient's symptomology severity, safety needs, his or her level of function, the condition of the support system, and at times the patient's motivation. There are immediate risks that indicate inpatient care is needed without looking at impairment. However,

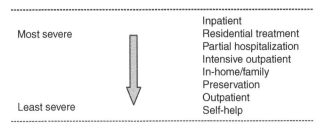

Figure 1.1 *The continuum of psychiatric services.*

when there is a potential safety risk, the patient's functional impairment is reviewed. Table 1.1 gives a general idea of the elements of function that are considered when making level-of-care assignments. Someone with severe impairment would logically meet the criteria for inpatient care or PHP based on the particular criteria, whereas someone with moderate or mild impairment might qualify for IOP.

The fluid and political nature of defining criteria makes it difficult to describe all IOP and PHP parameters; however, these programs ideally serve patients who meet some set of qualifying criteria. The patient who meets the criteria usually has less severe impairment of normal functioning in one or more of the areas.[1] However, this patient is not acute or symptomatic enough to be admitted to a psychiatric inpatient unit, but needs more help than a weekly counseling appointment. In many of these situations, the patient will be admitted as an inpatient if there is no clinical intervention at a lower level of care. The next section discusses how a patient's level of care is determined for PHP or IOP.

The Ideal

In ideal terms, the patient admitted to the PHP has more acute symptoms and is lower functioning than a patient in the IOP. The PHP patient is considered to need the services of a psychiatrist to evaluate appropriateness for medication and to start the patient on a trial of medication, if indicated. The psychiatrist is able to monitor for tolerance and side effects and increase medication as necessary. The PHP patient is present

---

[1] The term *baseline* is used interchangeably with *normal*. *Baseline* can refer to what is perceived to be a chronic patient's highest attainable level of functioning.

Table 1.1 *Functioning Criteria Used in Level-of-Care Decisions*

Criteria	Severe Impairment	Moderate Impairment	Mild Impairment
Hygiene	Unable to do	Must be reminded	Declining hygiene capability
Nutrition	Unable to do	Only with supervision	Declining diet
Daily tasks	Unable to do	Needs guidance	Declining ability
Ambulation	Nonambulatory	Only with assistance	—
Relationships	Withdrawn, terminated	Increased withdrawal	—
Abuse	Abused or abusing	—	—
Frustration/anger	—	Increased problems	—
Days since last workday	—	—	—
Work status	Five days since last day at work/10 since last day at school	—	—
Legal issues	Evicted/arrested	—	Arrested
Transportation	Does not have	Problems getting it	Not a problem
Ability to care for dependent	Unable to do	Threatened removal of children from home	Mild difficulty/child welfare involvement
Maintain household	Unable to do	Possible eviction/foreclosure	Late payments

longer during the programming day for more observation and will have more opportunity for learning coping skills. At the time of discharge, the PHP patient should step down either to the IOP level of care or to regular outpatient services.

Ideally, the IOP patient evidences milder symptomology and either needs more talk therapy or more coping skills education. The IOP patient is considered to be either less symptomatic or more stable than the PHP patient, but is not ready to step down to regular outpatient services. The IOP patient may be tolerating medication, but is waiting for medication effectiveness so as to be able to return to work or school, or be able to function on a given day without additional support. At the time of discharge, the IOP patient should go to outpatient services.

The Reality

As with almost all domains of life, the reality and ideal do not match. The incongruity between reality and the ideal in the PHP/IOP program frequently has to do with money and the criteria attached to funding sources. If it is not the money, it has to do with the dynamics of acuity, dysfunctional patient agendas, and the pitfalls of depending on the self-report of a patient who does not tell everything in the admitting department. The reality also means that the average PHP/IOP program will get an inappropriate referral from time to time, which can include:

- The malingerer avoiding work or school
- The drug-seeking patient only there to see the psychiatrist
- The geriatric patient with advanced dementia unable to participate
- The noncompliant, aggressive adolescent with an enabling parent
- The unmotivated, noncompliant addict referred by an employer

Patients and payer sources have various agendas, and IOP and PHP clinicians will have to respond as professionally as possible.

The Rules of the Money

If a hospital or organization has an insurance contract, whether governmental or private, it is contractually required to abide by the payer source's or managed care organization's (MCO's) admission and utilization policy and to treat the patient accordingly. If the payer source or MCO does not see a need for the admission and for continued stay, it will not pay. An MCO may only pay for IOP when it seems that the patient meets the criteria for PHP. A payer source may require frequent review, ask tangential questions, and only approve or certify a few days at a time. The more payer sources involved, the more sets of criteria for the IOP and PHP that require adherence.[2]

---

[2] Many doctors will stop accepting a managed care payer source if it has difficult credentialing, certification, and reimbursement procedures and low reimbursement rates.

Medicaid and Medicare are typically the pacesetters in the United States with regard to restrictive criteria. If there is a Medicare or Medicaid patient in the group, there are restrictions regarding the clinician credentials and group size. The payer sources may also require documentation to be in a particular form and that services be provided within a specified time frame. One payer source will accept one master's-level credential as billable, but not another. In addition, payer sources may require additional services or restrict the services that will be reimbursed.

Above all else, the rules of the money do not look at a patient's improvement. The standard for a patient to be admitted is determined in terms of acuity. A patient is usually allowed to stay in if he or she continues to present with acuity. However, some payer sources will invoke time limits and stop approving more days for an acute patient under the premise that the service is not appearing to benefit the patient.

The Dynamics of Acuity

A patient's symptomology or the acuity of the symptoms can be a dynamic, changing matter. A patient can crash in the short time between the intake assessment and admission to the program. A patient who presented as qualifying for PHP or IOP at the intake assessment may present as needing inpatient care when actually admitted to the program, even if it is only hours later. Depending on the payer source and the particular reviewer, the typical patient is admitted to the program based on the insurance company's willingness to pay. The psychiatrist seeing the patient or the program staff may see other symptoms that the patient did not present with or report the night before, which makes sending the patient from PHP or IOP to inpatient admittance a necessity.

On the other hand, PHP and IOP are used for step-down purposes from inpatient care, such as further stabilization, as long as a patient appears to be stable enough in the eyes of the payer source or MCO to leave inpatient care. The MCO has usually laid out what it will pay for and will suggest to the patient's psychiatrist a step-down to PHP or IOP. Regardless of the primary complaint leading to admission, the patient stepping down to PHP or IOP likely has started taking medication, has demonstrated tolerance of the medication, and has no further active suicidal ideation (and could contract for safety if still having some suicidal thoughts), but still the patient may present as very acute and fragile.

The patient may have times of fragility given that the recovery process is not a constant and steady trajectory. Instead, as depicted in Figure 1.2, the recovery process resembles a series of valleys and hills. The valleys mean that a patient will have a series of regressions and the hills indicate periods of improvement (or good days and bad days).

Some days the patient may seem more depressed or symptomatic than others. The patient may even be readmitted as an inpatient on a bad day. The bad days or periods may be related to medication effectiveness, medication compliance, substance use, and the introduction of stress, based on what happens or what the patient starts to process in the program. The bottom line is that psychiatric treatment takes time and may mean adjustments and changes in treatment as the patient's acuity and needs require.

Furthermore, acuity can breed acuity. A PHP/IOP program is intense largely because it has a variety of people with acute symptoms. One hopes the staff is seasoned and accustomed to the acuity; the patients are not. In a grand sense, the average patient is being exposed to information, emotion, and behavior that he or she does not deal with in normal life. This new information can distract the patient and trigger anxiety or a trauma reaction. In turn, the patient's treatment plan may have to be revised to address the newly identified acuity.

A realistic situation is that there are patients who come in with agendas that are not necessarily honest or realistic to the clinician and staff. There are patients who mask an addiction. There are malingering patients who try to get out of work or school. There are families that push elderly patients into treatment as a way of babysitting. There are attention-seeking patients who have the savvy to say what it takes to get into

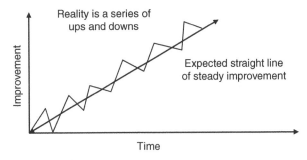

Figure 1.2 *The recovery process.*

treatment. It sometimes takes time for a clinician to determine whether a patient is either unmotivated or incapable to work on treatment.

To borrow from *Forrest Gump*, the reality of the PHP/IOP program is a lot like a box of chocolates. The program staff does not typically prescreen prospective patients and will not know how acute, motivated, compliant, or even aggressive the patient will be until they engage the patient. Furthermore, the program cannot decline patients in most situations. The staff has to react more to how the patients interact than be proactive. The PHP/IOP program milieu can change instantaneously based on the introduction of a disruptive patient or event.

THE ECOLOGY OF GAMES

Conceptualizing how to be successful in the intense and ever-changing PHP and IOP settings is a puzzle, if not a game. Regardless of patient assignment, acuity level, handling multiple tasks, and dealing with multiple actors and their multiple parameters seem to necessitate a number of so-called games that the clinician has to play. The games are not board games, nor are they like the manipulative or controlling interactions that some personality-disordered patients play with clinical staff and family.

Games Versus Gamey Behavior

In the clinical setting, the term *game* usually refers to manipulative, attention-seeking patient behavior, which creates drama (discussed more in Chapter 2) that annoys, stresses, and distracts clinical staff. The manipulative behavior can also distract other patients from focusing on their treatment. The manipulative behaviors can include:

- A patient leaving voice mails that report suicidal ideation with a plan and means who then does not answer the phone or door
- A patient making a tangential personal attack on a staff member for the staff member's "attitude"
- A patient making suicidal or homicidal comments and refusing to contract for safety

- A patient making distorted and embellished claims of victimhood
- A patient making a suicidal gesture by overdosing
- A patient twisting the words of staff back at a staff member
- A patient making different dramatic comments to staff
- A patient inciting other reactive patients to become angry

Whenever there is gamey behavior, the staff has to either rescue or control. After the crisis appears to be over, the patient tends to minimize what happened, blames the staff while claiming to be a victim, or places the blame on someone else.

Defining Games

However, in the case of this book, the term *game* is that suggested by Norton Long (1958). For Long, the game is a structured group activity in a particular territorial system. The game inherently gives the individual goals that define failure and success and how satisfaction will be gained. The game suggests roles and strategies in how the individual should perform the work. In Long's view, there is more than one game in a territory and they coexist.

Furthermore, these games are not trivial and cannot be taken lightly. The clinician should take these games seriously because they will lead to satisfaction in helping the patients and increase the value of the PHP/IOP program and the hospital or other agency to the community.

Understanding the different games that the clinician plays in the clinical context of the PHP and IOP programs will help to focus on the clinical activities that make a difference and lead to successful patient outcomes. These games also involve other patients, other departments, the doctors, colleagues, and other community organizations.

In the spirit of Long's theory, clinicians and teams develop excellence in PHP and IOP work by learning to play these games and refining how they play these games. The nature of clinical work is not typically measured quantitatively in terms of reaching a cumulative goal, but by the quality of service delivery. However, conceptualizing service delivery as a game allows for effective identification of meaningful metrics and standards because the game helps cue to the inherent goals and strategies that bring about success (Long, 1958, pp. 253–257).

ESSENTIAL PARADIGMS EVIDENT
THROUGHOUT IOP AND PHP SETTINGS

IOP and PHP settings with their different populations must operate differently in accordance with the treatment needs of the populations and the rules of the payer sources. Nevertheless, even with the variances found in different settings, there are two paradigms that are essential for playing the games: continuity and reasonable expectations.

Continuity

Continuity is another word for *continuation*, but it also implies connection and consistency. Continuity in various program elements helps a PHP/ IOP program to present as safe, stable, competent, and effective. Some primary program elements that require continuity include:

- Program schedule
- Patient rules/guidelines
- Team communication
- Educational material and delivery
- "Scripts" with patients, family, and others
- Documentation
- Treatment planning routines

Continuity does not mean a cookie-cutter approach to treatment. Each patient has different problems and varying needs, which dictate different treatment goals. However, those tasks and clinical services that can be routinized and consistently executed will allow reasonable individualization of treatment for a patient within time limitations and patient–professional boundaries.

Continuity is a must in PHP/IOP work, as both levels of care deliver services to groups and individuals simultaneously. Given the diversity of patients and the high level of acuity, if continuity as a value and principle is not maintained at its very basic level, there will be chaos, more safety risks, less patient satisfaction, fewer positive patient outcomes, and a poor reputation in the community. Without continuity, there is a higher risk of errors. Although there are numerous nuances in the games, it is highly unlikely that a clinician will encounter them all at once; they are intermittent and so there is a greater need for continuity to handle them.

On the flip side, continuity is a conceptual fence that can be put around a program. There are going to be personality-disordered patients who will engage in splitting between staff and other patients. The splitting can result in drama, loss of focus on treatment, and disruption in the therapeutic milieu. Commitment to practice continuity in its various aspects tends to illuminate the splitting and unites the team in appropriately responding to the splitting patient, while reducing the disruption of treatment to other patients. Continuity helps improve staff satisfaction, cohesion, and competency in handling more difficult and complex cases.

Continuity can also imply quality. While adults tend to express recognition and appreciation of quality more than children and adolescents do, the average patient coming to a PHP/IOP is a consumer wanting confidential and confident help with problems. Although patients are not experts on what it takes to deliver good service, they can tell when the program is a chaotic mess, unsafe, and unhelpful. On the other hand, the longer continuity is maintained in a particular direction, the better program elements can be refined and polished.

Reasonable Expectations

Continuity in the IOP and PHP settings is best sustained under reasonable expectations. In a grand sense, developing reasonable expectations is part of the professional growth process, but seems to escape most therapy textbooks. Although *reasonable* is a vague term in and of itself, within the PHP/IOP setting it means:

- There will be limits to the progress any one patient will likely make
- Acutely symptomatic patients are less capable of insight-based therapy
- Rarely will a PHP or IOP patient resolve all presenting problems
- Different patients benefit differently from different treatment modalities
- The recovery of different patients occurs at different paces
- Not all patients benefit from PHP or IOP

Consequences Without Reasonable Expectations

Numerous consequences can happen in the absence of reasonable expectations. The clinician sets inappropriate treatment goals. The clinician and team work harder than the patient. The interventions tend to be vague and nonspecific, if not idealistic. The patient does not feel satisfaction and neither does the staff. Furthermore, MCO utilization managers from outside the organization can make treatment mandates by phone and/or refuse to approve any more days, because the treatment does not seem to be effective and the patient gets discharged before the necessary progress is made.

Understanding Reasonable Expectations

Understanding reasonable expectations and limits arises out of trial and error in interacting with managed care and learning patient profiles. The MCOs make the decision in the end as to what is reasonable because they control the reimbursement, and MCOs can change what is considered reasonable without prior notice. Even as profiling has a negative connotation, it is evident that diagnoses in the medical textbooks and the *Diagnostic and Statistical Manual of Mental Disorders* (the *DSM* series) would not be possible if the same sets of symptoms had not been seen over and over again.[3] The clinician who is able to profile and to apply the profile becomes mindful of limits and reasonable expectations and becomes successful at playing the game. In a cognitive learning sense, the clinician in the IOP and PHP setting develops a schema of how profiles and MCO expectations match up to understanding reasonable expectations.

Being aware of limits and reasonable expectations should logically extend to what is going to be practical in treatment goals and interventions. For the PHP and IOP programs, this means limits in what they can do to help the patient improve in a number of areas. These areas of limitations include:

- The patient's level of crisis and motivation
- The patient's acuity and capability
- The level of family dysfunction

---

[3] The introduction of the *DSM-5* discusses the development of the *Diagnostic and Statistical Manual of Mental Disorders* and the collaborative revision process based on research findings (American Psychiatric Association, 2013, pp. 5–10).

- The time limitation imposed by the MCOs
- The clinician has limits and boundaries

Clinicians must appreciate these limitations as part of the ecology of games in order to act in practical and reasonable ways. Furthermore, these limitations fit within a tension between symptomology and capability where severity in symptomology means less capability. Table 1.2 illustrates this tension. At the severe end of symptomology, the patient cannot function and is capable of little. At the mild end of symptomology, the patient has little to no impairment in functioning. The Global Assessment of Functioning (GAF) scale, which is axis V on the historical, multiaxial diagnosis, has been a way of scoring this functioning.[4]

Table 1.2 *Tension of Symptomology and Capability*

Most Severe	None
Patient is preoccupied with trauma	Patient is not trauma focused
Cannot focus or engage	Focused and engaged
Cannot take care of self	No problem in performing ADLs[5]
No insight	Insightful
Will not take medication	Compliant with medication
Cannot interact	No problem interacting
Family is highly pathological	Family is very healthy
MCO gives significant time	MCO is giving minimal time
Clinician is new/green	Clinician is seasoned/experienced
Program design is not an appropriate fit	Program is an appropriate fit

---

[4] The *DSM-5* has discontinued use of the multiaxial system (American Psychiatric Assocation, 2013, p. 16). However, at the time of book preparation, MCOs in the United States have continued to require the multiaxial diagnosis for billing purposes. There does not appear to be a specific, announced date for cessation of use of the multiaxial diagnosis. Therefore, it will be an incremental migration in terms of actual practice.

[5] ADLs refer to *activities of daily living*, which include hygiene, cooking, bill-paying, balancing a checkbook, laundry, cleaning.

The capabilities of the clinician and the terms of the insurance policy also fit into the tension between symptomology and capability. If the clinician has developed the skill to identify and communicate accurately and effectively the patient's symptomology and functioning to the MCO, then in essence there is an inherent improvement in the patient's capability to recover. Also, if the clinician is skilled in educating the patient on appropriate goals according to the patient's functioning level, then also in essence there is improvement in a patient's ability to recover.

Another way of conceptualizing realistic expectations in PHP and IOP is the metaphor of the food-sorting mechanism used in produce and fishing operations. Although these devices are of different designs, the intent is that any food product (animal or vegetable) that is graded by size (such as an apple, orange, or live crab) falls through specific-sized spaces or is compared with standardized, sized models. The smaller sizes fall through and the larger sizes are moved on or are kept.

In this metaphor, the patients with the higher acuity or greater symptomology are the larger sized items. Patients with higher acuity and symptomology have the tendency to be unable to handle the more abstract, complex, and stressful matters. They are more likely to be unable to cope with the environment and may evidence panic attacks or other emotional breakdowns to comparatively small stressors. Conversely, the higher functioning person with less symptomology can handle increasing levels of complexity, environmental stimulation, and social stressors, and they fall through the holes or spaces.

Reasonable expectations also could be called conservative expectations or boundaries. In their states of depression and of being overwhelmed, patients frequently come in with idealistic and unrealistic expectations of wanting to address everything quickly. They want the pain to go away quickly and possibly expect antidepressants to work as fast as antibiotics. Many patients want to address abstract issues when they should be focusing on medical and behavior tasks, such as taking their medication, going for walks, and opening their window blinds.

In the different IOP and PHP cohorts, there is a consistent need to tell patients that the program will not likely help them recover completely, but that it should help them recover sufficiently to return to their normal lives and then they will likely continue their recovery in regular outpatient services. Patients also need information providing perspective about mental illness and how it prevents people from functioning.

Furthermore, it is important to lay out what is normal for a human being suffering from symptomology. From that point, it is appropriate to prioritize what is important to the patient and to guide treatment tasks that will address symptomology and contribute to recovery and fit those priorities.

Sometimes reasonable goals are already built into the medical record/documentation computer systems used by many hospitals. Many of the systems have approved goals that were determined by a committee or consultant to be best practices or even evidence based. For example, there are set goals in these systems for coping skills and symptom identification, triggers, and medication compliance. Going back to the concept of games, these computer systems with their supplied sets of goals give the clinician beginning clues of strategies and tasks to follow to be successful in delivering effective service to the PHP and IOP patients they serve.

OVERVIEW OF THE BOOK

Chapter 2: Understanding Team Work and Milieu in Partial Hospitalization and Intensive Outpatient Programs

This chapter discusses the ongoing cooperative game of providing a therapeutic milieu based on setting up and maintaining order and eschewing control as a goal. The game includes understanding and maintaining professional boundaries and relationships, the commitment to continuity, effective clinical communication with patients, and effective communication with psychiatrists and other departments.

Chapter 3: The Initial Treatment Plan

This chapter discusses the game of initial treatment planning. This is a game of joining with the patient in as little time as possible in a way that is adequately compassionate but sufficiently detached and that produces realistic treatment goals for the short treatment time allowed.

Chapter 4: Concurrent Treatment Planning

This chapter discusses the game of identifying treatment progress while documenting the necessary acuity to buy more treatment time from

MCOs. It includes a game plan for getting the right information for concurrent treatment planning. It also discusses cooperating with utilization review departments to get more reimbursed days of treatment from MCOs and participating when necessary in the dreaded peer-to-peer review.

Chapter 5: Discharge Planning

This chapter discusses the game of discharge planning. It includes dealing with the consideration of the different types of patients and psychiatrists. It also includes understanding the available aftercare resources.

Chapter 6: Group Therapy

This chapter discusses the game of group therapy as it is the primary treatment modality in the PHP/IOP setting. It outlines how to play this game in terms of facilitating an effective therapy group. It also discusses the limits of the group therapy modality at the PHP/IOP level of care compared to an outpatient therapy group. It also includes how to begin to run a group and how to deal with common group problems.

Chapter 7: Psychoeducation

This chapter discusses the game of providing psychoeducation. It discusses the purposes and suggested content of education. It also describes organizing a system for continuity in providing educational experiences.

Chapter 8: Safety Issues

This chapter discusses the game of safety and risk management. It includes a perspective on developing a safe milieu and dealing with suicidal and aggressive patients. It suggests a method for the clinician to use when making a protective services report and for maintaining relationships with patients and/or their families. Finally, it explores the safety issues pertaining to different subjects (sex, trauma, religion, and politics) and confidentiality.

Chapters 9, 10, 11, 12, and 13

Chapters 9 through 13 focus on working with the different cohorts and the application of the different games discussed in Chapters 2 to 8. Each chapter covers the use of the different treatment modalities, discharge planning, and unique problems of each cohort.

Chapters 14, 15, and 16

Chapters 14 through 16 discuss some of the recurring difficult situations and unique problems that occur in the PHP/IOP setting. These chapters suggest options for handling the situations in ways that minimize disruption to the milieu.

Chapter 14: The Borderline Personality–Disordered Patient

This chapter discusses the game of working with the borderline personality–disordered patient with the aim of providing appropriate service to the patient and simultaneously minimizing disruption to the program milieu. It focuses on working with the borderline personality–disordered patient in terms of joining, treatment planning, and handling the patient in group therapy and in the milieu.

Chapter 15: A Death in the Program

Deaths of patients in the PHP/IOP program do occur. There will be suicides and there will be natural deaths. This chapter briefly discusses a decision-making process and possible actions that staff can take when a patient dies.

Chapter 16: Problems With Colleagues and Other Departments

Problems do happen and this chapter discusses various types of problems that occur. Often, there are problems with psychiatrists and there are problems with departmental staff. Sometimes, there are staff members who are dysfunctional individuals themselves. Sometimes, there are problems with other hospital department employees. This chapter suggests options for action and coping with the unchangeable.

Chapter 17: Concluding Thoughts

This chapter provides a brief summary of the book. It offers some closing words of encouragement.

REFERENCES

American Psychiatric Association. (2013). *Diagnostic and statistical manual of mental disorders* (5th ed.). Arlington, VA: American Psychiatric Publishing.

Long, N. (1958). The local community as an ecology of games. *American Journal of Sociology, 64*, 251–261.

CHAPTER TWO

Understanding Team Work and Milieu in Partial Hospitalization and Intensive Outpatient Programs

*T*he therapeutic milieu of the partial hospitalization program (PHP)/ intensive outpatient program (IOP) is a vital backdrop for the psychopharmacology and the group therapy. However, the milieu is often an afterthought because the focuses are therapy, patient safety, and managed care information requirements. However, adult patients will not stay, and child/adolescent patients will be more likely to act out if they do not feel safe. Patients must feel accepted and safe in the milieu if they are going to make themselves vulnerable, which they must do to participate in therapy. A therapeutic milieu at the PHP/IOP level is thus, in and of itself, a product or service.

The therapeutic milieu is not a coincidence, but is a cooperative venture. No one staff member can assume total responsibility for the milieu's therapeutic qualities, but each team member influences the milieu as a whole. If one team member is not in agreement with regard to the milieu, the quality, credibility, effectiveness, and productivity of the program are all at risk.

This chapter aims to help the reader understand the game of the therapeutic milieu in the PHP/IOP setting and identify ways to implement it. It discusses drama's threat to the order of the milieu and how to minimize it. It discusses the paradigm of order over control. It lays out the games that develop and maintain a PHP/IOP therapeutic milieu across the different patient cohorts.

MILIEU DEFINED

A *milieu* is typically defined as an environment or culture. The therapeutic milieu has been considered an important element in psychiatric treatment for decades. There is no shortage of scholarly writing on the therapeutic milieu, but in maintaining fidelity to the body of work on partial hospitalization, DiBella, Weitz, Poynter-Berg, and Yurmark (1982) suggested that:

> A therapeutic milieu is a group treatment environment which is supervised and initially designed by appropriate professionals; it provides a model of the everyday world of reality and maximized opportunities for patients to benefit from their social and physical surroundings. (p. 66)

DiBella and colleagues (1982, p. 66) identified the following seven necessary elements of a therapeutic milieu in a PHP:

1. The milieu is a priority over any one particular therapy.
2. Group therapy is used.
3. Patients have some responsibility for the milieu.
4. Problem solving should be achieved through community consensus rather than by a few authority figures.
5. The community should meet to discuss information and interactions that apply to both the staff and the patients.
6. There is accountability to a governing body.
7. As many milieu events as possible should facilitate patient success in the community.

The treatment model that DiBella and colleagues followed in New York was a program that lasted most of the day, which allowed time for inclusion of the seven elements.

THE MILIEU AS AN ECONOMY

However, in the 30 years since DiBella and his coauthors wrote their book, managed care has shortened the program day, program week, and patient length of stay. Although Medicaid-funded child and adolescent programs tend to have more time each day to foster an intentional community, there is little time for the inclusion of all the aforementioned milieu elements in adult programs. As noted earlier, the focus in most PHPs/IOPs is not the milieu but the delivery of billable services and documentation of patient symptomology in accordance with the managed care requirements and productivity standards.

Compared to inpatient services, managed care has in essence changed the nature of the milieu in the PHP/IOP setting from being an environment to being an economy with multiple actors and inputs. The milieu of the inpatient or residential treatment unit is under the 24-hour supervision of the nurses and/or staff and can maintain the rubric of an environment.[1] The staff literally holds the keys to the doors, which means control of the milieu environment inputs and outputs within the legal frameworks of program policy and patient rights. The group of patients stays together in the confined space behind those doors. The nurses and/or staff administer the program schedule and then monitor and adjust the milieu environment as necessary according to how the group of patients is behaving.[2]

As an economy in the managed care environment, the staff at best has an influence as an actor in the PHP/IOP milieu that extends beyond the unit doors and beyond the control of the staff. Many patients leave the program site and interact with each other outside of program hours. Patient behavior or patient events off the program site, whether off the unit or off grounds, can have an immense effect on the milieu. Such behavior and events include fraternization, sexual relationships, cohabitation, patient suicide/suicide attempts, natural death of patients, conflict among patients, and other patient crises. Staff members cannot exert the same level of influence over the milieu as inpatient or residential staff, but they can be dominant and influential economic actors who knowledgeably play the appropriate game using its objectives and strategies.

PHP/IOP staff must be mindful of the tension of supply and demand. The patients, payer sources, and the staff are all economic actors. Regardless of the situation, the patients are voluntary consumers of the services and generally can choose whether to attend or be absent. The patient may also reject the clinical staff's recommendations or become dissatisfied and not return. As is discussed further in Chapter 4, the managed care organization (MCO), which is the patient's payer source, is also a consumer alongside the patient. The MCO can contractually dictate the supply of certain services and clinical information. The MCO may

---

[1] The program model does vary, but it is typical that the inpatient hospital unit is managed by nursing staff. The residential program is typically managed by master's- or doctoral-level counselors/therapists.

[2] This can mean transferring or discharging noncompliant or disruptive patients based on the circumstances.

also deny payment for certain services that are a normal part of the program design. If the patient is not attending, the required service is not delivered, or the required clinical information is not supplied, the MCO will decertify and not pay for any more services. The MCO utilization reviewer may still decertify despite best efforts, and the patient will be abruptly discharged, possibly affecting the milieu. The PHP/IOP staff is very much a supplier of a number of economic goods and services and must seek to be influential rather than act authoritatively.

Understanding the influence in the economy begins with observing that a typical, non–treatment-savvy patient entering a PHP or IOP is anxious and wary of coming to a stigmatic place in a time of crisis and would rather not be there. The patient is motivated enough to be there by the expectation that his or her symptoms and distress will be eliminated. The milieu as an economy should present itself as a refuge that is a safe, peaceful, and an empathetic setting to motivate a patient to engage in treatment and comply with treatment recommendations. It should maximize the patient's dignity and give the patient hope, which means talking to adult patients as if they are adults and not as children.[3] There is an inherent assumption that the vulnerable and anxious patient will be handled gently, but the average psychiatric patient needs to be talked to as a normal person. It is a challenge to create a stable and comfortable milieu that can be what the anxious patient needs.[4]

THE NORMAL PHP/IOP MILIEU

Even though the goal of treatment is stabilization of any patient who comes through the door, the ironic challenge is that the situation lends itself to anything but stability. In addition to the economy metaphor, and contrary to what DiBella and others suggest, the IOP and PHP milieu is normally an intense setting that is not representative of the everyday world. The IOP or PHP is an intentional destination for patients in states

---

[3] This is based on the concept of transactional analysis. Talking to a patient as an adult means talking to another adult friend or talking like an adult salesperson might talk to an adult customer in a sales situation.

[4] Many cluster-B personality-disordered patients (and parents of child patients) can be anxious to the point of being fragile, regardless of how the therapist approaches them.

of crisis, unstable mood, and diminished judgment, which leads to a reactive staff vigilance for high levels of acuity whether it be from personality disorder, suicidality, homicidal ideation, or psychosis. Depending on the assessment and admission processes, the staff never knows what clinical pathology and/or symptomology will come through the program door, making for discomfort and distress. Depending on the composition of the patient population, the emotional energy that arises out of the acuity can intensify and destabilize the milieu at any given time. The average, non–treatment-savvy PHP or IOP patient does not expect this intensity of the milieu and may complain or just not come back due to anxiety and an inability to tolerate the stress of the milieu.

Such intensity can make a PHP/IOP milieu evolve into a group of insensitive survivors. Survivors exhibit those behaviors to endure a difficult situation. Staff and management can be overwhelmed,[5] guarded, cold, vigilant, and rigid (if not insensitive) while trying to do their jobs. The fragile patients may survive in the intense milieu and chaos by withdrawing and either avoiding or being reluctant to talk about personal issues in therapy groups. Personality-disordered patients may drive the milieu intensity with tales of crisis and trauma, but complain simultaneously about the lack of peace. The intensity can be a further reinforcement of such survivor behavior, which may degrade both the milieu's overall therapeutic and economic value and stunt the capacity of the milieu to grow in size and accommodate more patients.

Also, the intensity can precipitate frequent milieu disruptions when there are one or more difficult patients who are reactive, labile, intolerant, and behaving immaturely. Many acute and personality-disordered patients are insensitive and do not tolerate the diversity and acuity of other patients. Some patients act entitled and demanding. Some are judgmental, verbally abusive, and aggressive toward staff and other patients. Some patients in a manic or psychotic state make inappropriate, aggressive,[6] and impulsive statements to other patients and staff. If unchecked and unaddressed, such clinical phenomena create a chilling effect and a

---

[5] This staff behavior could also be identified as burnout or emotional impairment.

[6] Defensiveness and aggressiveness are often confused because they both come across as angry. Assessing both the context and the content of the patient's behavior is crucial to making an appropriate response to the patient.

chaotic milieu and reduce attendance the next day, in turn reducing revenue and productivity.

In addition to clinical symptoms, patient revolt can create intense drama and chaos in the milieu and reduce its therapeutic effectiveness. Many depressed patients may have higher levels of irritability and anxiety, which causes patients to argue, throw tantrums, or even fight. A patient can brazenly criticize a therapist out in the open or exhibit passive-aggression by instigating drama.

DEFINING *DRAMA*

Drama is a three-way form of communication that is commonly depicted in a triangle as in Figure 2.1. Drama has three roles: the victim, the perpetrator, and the rescuer. The roles in drama are interchangeable, as all three people can exchange the roles with each other (examples: victim becomes rescuer, rescuer becomes perpetrator, and perpetrator becomes the victim).

Drama is an immature, passive-aggressive form of communication of emotion and not fact.

Drama also can be a power move to control others by dividing and conquering. This power move is also called "splitting." Someone who either claims to be a victim or rescuer makes a third person out to be a perpetrator. The person claiming to be a rescuer or a victim attempts to portray legitimate moral power through self-righteous anger or confusion. If he or she demonstrates self-righteous anger or confusion, the assumption is that the alleged perpetrator has failed or has hurt the identified victim. It is held here that when it comes to the initiation of drama,

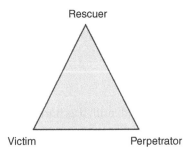

Figure 2.1 *The triangle of drama.*

the one first communicating victimhood tends to be the actual, initial perpetrator.[7]

Many personality-disordered patients and patients who come from chaotically enmeshed families reenact drama because it is a habit. They distort and embellish the behavior of their family members while minimizing their own contributions to drama. Instigating drama could also be a maladaptive coping mechanism that patients use to avoid facing their responsibility for their own issues. Such patients instigate drama the way their families normally do, but drama is a counterproductive force in psychiatric treatment, especially treatment that is supposed to be time limited. It interferes with both the work of the staff and the treatment of other patients.

In the PHP/IOP setting, the instigation of drama typically comes in the form of a patient making a statement that has the potential to "split" two or more staff members.[8] This split has the potential of setting staff in conflict with each other. The typical, instigating patient will make a critical, emotional judgment that embellishes or distorts reality. Such distortions have a modicum of truth, but often misrepresent the original context. In some cases, the patient projects or blames the staff member for something the patient actually says or does (this is called *projection*). The patient claims to be a victim of a staff member or a rescuer of other patients.

The following scenario illustrates the victimhood role in drama. A new patient named Nancy goes to Susan, the nurse, and says that she wants a new social worker because Dave, her assigned social worker, is too pushy and not patient enough with her, and Nancy thinks Dave is mad at her. Furthermore, Nancy claims that Dave does not care about her problems. Interpretation: Nancy is claiming she is a victim of Dave and is asking for Susan to rescue her.[9]

---

[7] The one claiming to be a victim is often attempting to punish the alleged perpetrator. The one claiming to be a rescuer often is projecting emotion onto a perceived victim or is trying to make the identified victim retaliate toward the alleged perpetrator.

[8] Other examples of drama instigation include staff splitting other staff and family members starting drama. Even other agency/hospital staff members from outside the department who interface with the department or patients can instigate drama.

[9] Note that Nancy is making no specific factual statements of any behavior.

The following scenario illustrates the rescuer instigating the drama. A patient named Sam goes to another social worker and claims that other people are bothered by what Dave, the social worker, had said in a group. Sam said that he is embarrassed for the rest of the group. Interpretation: Sam is claiming that Dave is the perpetrator and others are the victims.[10]

If the staff members on the receiving end of the "split," or complaint, have a agenda to exert control in the department or are highly anxious themselves or have low emotional intelligence, they tend to get pulled into the drama and undermine the staff member who was made out to be the perpetrator. The clinician or other staff member pulled into the complaint usually tries to rescue the complaining patient and violates patient–staff boundaries and boundaries among staff, and in turn becomes a perpetrator. A staff member who is either green or who has low emotional intelligence is prone to getting pulled into the patient drama.

A subgroup of patients such as the shadow group (see the following text) can become enmeshed and sabotage the group therapy dynamics. The subgroup can target a specific patient or staff member for a panoply of reasons. Patients enabled to instigate drama can end up controlling the department, dictating treatment, monopolizing group therapy, and undermining other patients' treatment. Depending on the composition of the patient population, there will be some inherent power games against staff by one or more patients.

The "shadow group" phenomenon is a frequent and prevalent subgroup occurrence that is reflective of the economy paradigm and a source of drama. The shadow group is two or more patients who become enmeshed with each other in such a way that they demonstrably put the enmeshed relationships above their roles as individual patients in the program.[11] The shadow group will vary in size and influence, based on the composition of the patient population. The shadow group members become emotionally dependent on each other and become junior therapists to each other even to the point of eschewing the clinician. They often intrude into each other's personal affairs, forgetting that they are the patients with their own individual clinical needs and their own, individual, diminished functioning levels. The shadow group tends to come

---

[10] In reality, Sam is actually projecting his own emotion on the other patients.

[11] The shadow group tends to attract individuals with personality-disorder traits or codependent traits.

back late from breaks and tends to make its disclosures outside of formal group sessions (and do group therapy outside of the program parameters) often to the point where treatment progress is difficult to monitor and often impeded. The shadow group tends to demonstrate group contagion (Redl & Wineman, 1957), where the group can quickly rise up in anger and scapegoat a therapist or another patient in unison. Regardless of staff and therapist variables, the shadow group can seriously impair the therapeutic value of the milieu.

In light of the potential chaos and disruptive phenomena, maintaining the milieu requires intentionality and mindfulness. The milieu as an economy is highly complex, and accepting the magnitude is crucial. Although all milieu variables and details cannot be covered, and each team must work out how to play the game for itself, there are some common strategic starting points for milieu development. These strategic starting points are mind-sets and paradigms defining who the patients tend to be and how a professional team acts.

THE GAME OF THE MILIEU

Therefore, the game makes the milieu therapeutic through commitment to the appropriate strategies; commitment to standards; commitment to routinizing the mundane, recurring tasks; and commitment to maintaining the necessary elements. Together, these commitments should create a PHP and/or IOP therapeutic milieu that assists the individual patients in both focusing on and meeting their individual treatment goals. The structured portions of the milieu should provide some slack or shock absorption that compensates when there is a disruption in another part of the economy. Although not all of these are discussed in detail, the elements of a PHP/IOP milieu as an economy could include:

- The maintenance of the facility
- The layout of the facility
- The cleanliness of the facility
- The lighting of the facility
- The type of furniture and its condition
- The degree to which the facility uses updated technology
- The admitting processes
- The formal policies communicated in writing

- The daily operational processes
- The quality of the printed materials
- The program schedule
- The development and refinement of the educational program
- The presence of food service and rules regarding food and beverage consumption in the program
- The punctuality of the staff
- The regular attendance of staff at their scheduled work times
- The emotional states and attitudes of the staff (including anger management)
- The interpersonal relationships among staff
- The communication among staff
- The consistency of staff in communicating and enforcing policies and schedules
- The ability of the management to lead
- The clinical insight of the manager/director
- The philosophy, management style, priorities, and attitude of the management
- The cooperation or lack of cooperation among staff (including doctors)
- The manner in which the staff handles crises
- The manner in which the staff handles difficult patients
- The way patients behave toward the staff
- The way the staff acts toward patients
- The boundaries the staff have with patients and each other
- The way patients act toward each other inside and outside of program hours (often developing a "shadow" group)

Paradigms and Mind-Sets

Because of the nature of the service, developing and maintaining a milieu are ongoing processes and can never be a complete and finished product; the game paradigm has benefits for conceptualizing strategies. Reasonable expectations are intertwined throughout the paradigms and mind-sets of the development and maintenance of a milieu. The staff must cooperatively engage in the tasks and strategies to make the milieu therapeutic and maintain it as such. By envisioning playing the game as a team, the staff members are able to develop common strategies and tasks that work for them as a team and help meet their different objectives.

The staff must be mindful of the necessary strategies needed to maintain the milieu. Contrary to the findings of DiBella and colleagues, although the clinical needs of the patients are the focus of treatment, the patients are not in charge of the milieu. PHP and IOP patients are temporary milieu members seeking the professional services of the staff. The patients should be focused on their own symptoms that are disrupting their lives,[12] and the staff should play the game with its inherent tasks and strategies around the periphery of the patients. The basic strategies of the game include order and not control, routinization in all possible situations, drama management, and adult-level communication.

The Strategy of Order and Not Control

The overall strategy that the staff must use to structure and maintain a therapeutic milieu is *order* and not *control*. The agreement on order is either coincidental or mindful. Order is a larger construct that is created by two or more individuals who agree and have trust among themselves. Order is very much a cooperative and unifying venture. It requires two or more people to agree to roles that are in their common interest and appreciate the significance of those roles. Cooperating to maintain order will create benefit, reduce the likelihood of negative consequences, or reduce the severity of unavoidable consequences. In the PHP/IOP setting, the effects of maintaining order affect both the staff and the patients.

In adhering to a strategy of maintaining order, the team agrees and cooperates on a course of action that will be reasonable to implement and sustain. The strategy also includes the recognition of boundaries and roles. The strategy of maintaining order means routine communication practices about relevant patient information and group dynamics. The act of agreeing and carrying out the course of action is the larger part of the game. Order also requires a sense of faith or fidelity and trust. Staff members who do not show fidelity and trust will inherently sabotage the game of order. If staff members do not cooperate in maintaining order in the milieu, it can become quickly evident through staff drama and

---

[12] Sometimes "treatment-savvy" patients know the games and may have manipulative agendas.

when a disruptive patient causes extended drama through multiple or extended staff splitting.

In contrast, control in and of itself in a milieu is impossible. Trying to control others in a therapeutic milieu means that you are seeking to dominate others and restrain your patients in some form or fashion. The motivation to control is individual and emotional versus logical and team focused. The motivation for control is either anger or insecurity, where the controlling behavior is expected to meet the emotional need of the one seeking control. In its very nature, the pursuit of control over others is not therapeutic as it assumes no limits or boundaries. The strive for control ends up in divisive struggles and emotionally immature expressions that distract the team members from focusing on the delivery of services.[13] Control is secretive and puzzling, but order is well communicated and clearly understood. Control games quite often lead to chaos and high staff turnover[14] because no one wants to be controlled by anyone else.

Subscribing to Order

Probably the best way to think about order is *subscribing* to order. This is a useful strategy when communicating with difficult and manipulative patients who may make demands or complaints. Appealing to order is logical, rational, and done with calmness. Although there is no guarantee that the patient will be convinced to comply with treatment, not appealing to order usually puts the professional staff in an undesirable and non-therapeutic emotional power struggle that could have been avoidable.[15]

---

[13] Micromanagement is a supervisory behavior that emanates from anxiety and presents as a pursuit of control. The supervisor or manager gives little to no decision-making power to otherwise-qualified professional staff. This behavior is highly present in the mental health and social service fields.

[14] Micromanagement is a typical expression of control. In micromanagement in the clinical situation, the supervisor, manager, or director allows little to no decision-making autonomy to clinicians. The micromanager requires his or her clearance or approval for routine decisions and tends to undermine any perception of a staff member demonstrating autonomy. In intense situations with high patient census and high acuity, micromanagement can engender drama.

[15] The challenging patient often tries to cast things in terms of a personal vendetta and makes the complaint as a personal attack.

In subscribing to order, a staff member demonstrates clinical principles and standards and recognizes that the program exists within a larger structure, which guides and puts limits on the program. The limits are organization policies, MCO utilization review, governmental authorities, accreditation, and societal norms and mores. There is a reason we do what we do and why we do it—everything is purposeful and can be explained.

Order is a constant where, hopefully, the patient sees how the program works and how he or she should expect treatment to be conducted. Order is very much about reducing the opportunity for personalized protests by patients who project entitlement or claim victimhood. Order also takes the heat off any one staff member who may come under fire by a patient or a clique of patients as an object of anger.

A Case Example

Nancy is a 33-year-old White female who was referred by her employee assistance program (EAP) for addiction treatment after she tested positive for cocaine. Nancy had attendance problems and was missing IOP sessions. Because hers was a managed care case, she was discharged twice for noncompliance, but came back through the admitting office within a day after discharge. Nancy did not respond to the phone calls of the drug–alcohol counselor, but came in after the second discharge and angrily accused the drug–alcohol counselor of having a personal vendetta against her.

Prior to the interaction, the supervisor got the background from the counselor and proceeded as follows:

Supervisor: Hi, I'm Dave. What can I do for you?

Nancy: Joyce kicked me out of the program.

Supervisor: Kicked you out of the program? What do you understand to be the reason?

Nancy: She said I wasn't coming to the program.

Supervisor: You weren't coming. Is there any truth to that?

Nancy: Well, yeah, but she shouldn't have discharged me.

Supervisor: The program is voluntary, but I understand that you came right back to admitting right after discharge. What brought you back?

Nancy: I have to be here for my job.

Supervisor: Who is requiring you to be here?

Nancy: My EAP makes me be here.

Supervisor: Okay . . . there's an EAP involved. With an EAP the rules are different. They will want a letter saying you complied with treatment, and I bet you will have to do a drug screen to get back on your work site. What makes it even more difficult is if you don't attend, your insurance will tell us to discharge you. We want to help you get back to work, but that will require you to attend the program so your insurance pays for you to be here and we can then report that you complied with treatment.

Nancy was irritable during the conversation, but afterward she was treatment compliant and completed the program. By subscribing to the order and giving some information about the insurance and EAP parameters, the supervisor was able to reframe the matter in terms of the order and remove a lot of emotion. The supervisor's subscribing to the order supported Joyce, the clinician's, credibility in the milieu even though Nancy still made subtle innuendoes of contempt for Joyce for the rest of Nancy's time in the program.

The Strategy of Routinization

Routine generally connotes boredom, insensitivity, and inflexibility, but it also suggests the essence of order and stability. Order is longitudinally demonstrated by the existence of a routine, both in an individual sense and in a group sense. In terms of a therapeutic milieu, the average unstable patient will likely embrace the routine before getting oriented to all of the rules. Therefore, the routine should be a smooth demonstration of order as it goes through the sequence or schedule of events. This section gives a theoretical basis of the development and maintenance of routine followed by some general areas of application.

Routine is the approach or attitude in which the milieu elements are maintained. The numerous elements necessitate using Adam Smith's "division of labor." Smith (1776/1977) noted that dividing up the tasks of production improved quality and produced more pins faster. With time and commitment, routinization can increase the efficiency with which elements are provided. The pursuit of routine can lead to identification of the milieu elements that are present in the particular situation or setting. Routinization can also increase the quality and refinement of those elements.

Routinization assumes that not all tasks must be created fresh over and over again. There are many tasks that will be required repeatedly. Trying to recreate them each time is inefficient.[16] The energy used to recreate tasks reduces the opportunity to address the unique situations that arise in the milieu. Assuming there are tight staffing patterns with little to no budget for clerical or administrative staff, the demands to create the milieu elements uniquely each time will detract from patient care and reduce the number of patients that can be accommodated.

Therefore, the higher the degree of routinization, the more likely the milieu can accommodate that maximum number of patients, which will lead to increased revenue. Once developed, a polished and refined routine can be repeated with increasing speed and less effort.

Routinization can also enable the milieu to be more stable when there are threats of disruptions or actual disruptions. Staff can devote more energy and attention to address disruptions because they spend less energy on the provision of the milieu elements. Furthermore, routinization can divide responsibility among staff to address issues and disruptions.

Routine and routinization can have a negative connotation when one considers that different patients have different needs. When a particular staff member has control issues, the different needs of different patients are often overemphasized as an argument against complying with routinization of program elements. However, taken to its logical end, none of the patients coming into a PHP or IOP have exactly the same needs because the patients are different people with different life situations. Trying to adapt to all patient differences is a futile endeavor and will inhibit ordering the milieu and might create unproductive chaos. Conversely, the modality of group therapy, which is discussed more in Chapter 6, has a normative tendency to find commonalities among patients. The reality is that the milieu

---

[16] Periodic review of the elements can be helpful and may indicate that changes should be made to increase effectiveness, but to maintain the milieu, frequent change should be avoided.

requires order, and routine is needed to maintain order. The hesitant or rogue staff member should at least be encouraged to contribute to the creation of the routine as a positive option and be allowed to shape the routines, but in turn must be held accountable to abide by the routine.[17]

The Strategy of Drama Management

Drama is a recurring challenge to the order of the milieu in a PHP/IOP. Drama is an unstable and immature form of communication. Drama causes chaos and distracts both patients and staff from focus on treatment and the tasks. Drama can ruin the program reputation. Inappropriate management of drama hurts staff morale. Left unchecked, drama leads to a hostile workplace that reduces productivity and increases safety risk and liability.

Despite its consequences, drama does happen in PHP/IOP settings. Furthermore, in every new job or practice situation, experiencing drama and how your new coworkers and manager or director address that drama evidences to be a rite of initiation. Very often, the staff member learns the weaknesses and problems of the current work situation and possibly the reason his or her predecessor left the job. Given the goal of maintaining order, *drama management* is the best mind-set to have and best clinical strategy to use when dealing with drama.

Elements of a Drama Management Policy

Given that clinicians do make mistakes, and true problems such as misconduct do happen, each patient should be heard in the name of patient safety and good risk management, but in support of the team it is essential to be fair when reviewing the facts of the dispute. It is poor judgment to assume that the clinician is automatically wrong, and when a patient makes a vague, emotional comment based on no specific fact, it is evident

---

[17] In terms of quality assurance, it is possible to measure the maintenance of order. All of the strategies for maintaining order can be operationalized as variables. Many of the variables of order are already measured through existing patient satisfaction tools that many hospitals purchase from outside vendors. Instruments can be created for measuring efforts to maintain order and tracked in a spreadsheet program.

that the patient is instigating drama. It is also demoralizing for the staff when the management does not provide some filter of perspective and consideration in such situations. A hostile workplace can evolve when a manager or director does not stand behind staff members when sociopathic, manipulative, and treatment-savvy patients approach with passive-aggressive attacks on line staff members.

Therefore, it is recommended that there be a mutually understood protocol, if not a written policy, for how staff and management will respond to the following situations:

- A patient requests a different social worker
- A patient claims to be a spokesperson for the rest of the group
- A patient makes a vague complaint that a social worker or clinician is not as patient or good as another social worker
- A patient complains about another patient
- A patient is uncomfortable with something a social worker said
- A patient claims that a social worker was mad, rude, inpatient, or insensitive
- A patient requests to go to a different group
- A patient requests a different doctor

The protocol should include:

- A script of what is to be said to the complaining patient
- Steps that will be adhered to by each staff member
- The role the supervisor will play, if any
- When risk management will be called
- When the patient will be referred back to the social worker/when the patient is complaining about needing help with something
- What kind of factual feedback will be given to line staff in such situations?[18]

The drama management protocol needs to be broad in nature to exhibit more of a philosophy of maintaining order than trying to cover every possible scenario.

---

[18] What the patient said should be factually stated. It is disruptive to say what the patient felt. Statement of feeling only engenders drama.

The Strategy of Adult-Level Communication

The manner in which drama and the PHP/IOP milieu are managed depends on the level of communication of staff and management. The communication that takes place in a PHP/IOP milieu is intended to take place within the order for specific treatment purposes. The order assumes that the therapist–staff relationship is a time-limited one with certain boundaries. The staff communication and reaction are expected to be in accordance with accepted standards of rational thinking, clinical judgment, and theory.

Much of the literature about patient–professional communication in psychiatric treatment covers what happens in the context of the formal setting of the therapy session, but the difference in the milieu is that there is a combination of informal and formal settings. With the opportunity of including multiple individuals, the informal setting provides a greater risk for drama and the problematic patient acting out and disrupting the milieu. Communication in both the formal and informal settings is the most pervasive staff input into the economy of the milieu.

In economic terms, staff communication presents as an opportunity or risk to produce various externalities and exchanges. The utterances of the staff can either calm the milieu and maintain order or stir it up and engender chaos. Staff either will feed into the emotional lability of patients or will respond in a manner that order is maintained and chaos is neutralized.

The communication from staff to patients should be that of modified empathy. The staff member needs to have emotional intelligence to demonstrate this. The communication by the staff should recognize and attend to the emotion of the patient, but observe rational emotional and behavioral limits. Emotion is irrational in and of itself, and it has both valid and invalid triggers. In this context, "unmodified empathy" assumes that the emotion is the message regardless of the validity of the trigger. In the intense setting of the PHP/IOP milieu, the emotion is frequently intense, and the staff member without emotional intelligence is at grave risk of crossing emotional boundaries and taking inappropriate ownership of patient issues and entering into a dramatic pattern of communication.

Emotional intelligence includes self-awareness, self-regulation, social skill, and empathy and motivation (Goleman, 1995). Clinicians generally have the empathy and motivation, but they often lack the self-awareness and self-regulation.

Self-regulation refers to the clinician having insight and evaluating in logical terms about where the patient is coming from and what may be motivating his or her behavior? The patient is likely to be in an elevated emotional state, and the job of the staff member and/or clinician is to be empathetic, calm and rational, and firm yet gentle. The nature of the clinician–/staff–patient interaction is ideally a complementary one in which the clinician is able to attend and respond in one of several ways that indicate that he or she has heard the patient and appreciated the patient's emotional state, but is mindful of the professional stance required in such a situation. The professional stance is of course an adult stance.[19]

What does it mean to have an adult stance? In the context of his transactional analysis approach, Berne (1964/2004) offers an objective idea. In Berne's approach, there are three ego (or emotional) states: parent, child, and adult. For Berne:

An ego state may be described phenomenologically as a coherent system of feelings related to a given subject, and operationally as a set of coherent behavior patterns; or pragmatically, as a system of feelings which motivates a related set of behavior patterns. (p. 23)[20]

A child has poor self-control and is immature, emotional, and reactive to negative or irritating phenomena (in other words, has poor coping skills). A parent tends to talk down in a didactic or teaching fashion with the intent of controlling or directing the child in the presence of negative phenomena. In Berne's framework, the adult demonstrates self-control, self-regulation, and rational thinking when dealing with negative situations. The adult stance, with its calm tone of voice, should calm down those situations in which the tension is thick enough to cut with a knife by providing dignity to the broken, crying patient.

Taking this full circle, the game of the milieu requires the strategy of the adult stance and adult level of communication. Creating an orderly milieu requires the logical stance of the adult ego state and its associated level of communication. There is no exception when difficult,

---

[19] This concept could apply to dealing with coworkers or colleagues. The reality in any work situation and professional field is that there are colleagues with poor emotional intelligence. More about this is discussed in Chapter 16.

[20] The page number for this quote varies with the edition.

personality-disordered, and immature patients come through the door of the program seeking attention and causing disruption. When professionals act immaturely and emotionally in reaction to immature patients, boundaries are crossed and chaos or drama between patients and staff ensues. The adult state is a very powerful state used to illuminate (or neutralize) the immature behavior and maintain order.[21]

In a behavioral sense, the strategy of adult communication can be operationalized by identifying scripts that a mature professional uses. The scripts include words, tone of voice, and voice inflection for situations and encounters. The script includes that the professional be calm and set limits, saying, "I will help you if I can" and "I will give you an answer if I know." The strategy of adult communication is mastered over time with practice, polish, and a desire to improve.

CONCLUSIONS

This chapter conceptualized the therapeutic milieu in the PHP/IOP as a game with goals and inherent strategies and explored the strategies used to play the games. The therapeutic milieu is that environment or backdrop of safety that patients need for productive therapy. Conceptualizing the PHP/IOP milieu as an economy illuminates the salient threats and assists in identification of the strategies and goals used to create and maintain safety.

The game of the milieu is complex and requires team attention to many elements. Because of this complexity, the milieu must be managed through strategies in the forms of mind-sets and paradigms. Team members subscribing to the maintenance of order in the milieu versus an attempt to control the milieu will engender a sense of fairness and stability when dealing with disruptive patients. Routinization arises out of the

---

[21] A professional is expected to be adult and rational in his or her approach, letting feelings be informed by logic and to set emotional boundaries. Making jokes or insensitive comments about patients happens everywhere, but it endangers the milieu. Furthermore, when supervisors and staff members complain behind each other's backs, the synergy needed to maintain the milieu is corrupted. In line with this, Section 2.01 of the National Association of Social Workers (NASW) *Code of Ethics* expects social workers to treat colleagues with respect (http://www.socialworkers.org/pubs/code/code.asp).

desire to create order and consistency in as many milieu elements as possible so as to free up energy and time to address clinical crises and milieu disruptions. Drama management is a suggested mind-set or philosophy to use in recognizing that some patients do instigate drama, causing its disruptive impact on the milieu; the therapy of other patients can be enhanced or minimized depending on the specific ways in which the staff responds to the drama. Adult communication following in the tradition of Berne's (1964/2004) system of transactional analysis is a behavioral mark of the professional treatment team seeking to influence the milieu in stable and therapeutic ways. The therapeutic milieu in a PHP/IOP is intense and engrossing.

REFERENCES

Berne, E. (2004). *Games people play*. New York, NY: Ballantine Books. (Original work published 1964)

DiBella, G., Weitz, G., Poynter-Berg, D., & Yurmark, J. L. (1982). *Handbook of partial hospitalization*. New York, NY: Brunner/Mazel.

Goleman, D. (1995). *Emotional intelligence*. New York, NY: Bantam Dell.

Redl, F., & Wineman, D. (1957). *The aggressive child. I: Children who hate: The disorganization and breakdown of behavior controls. II: Controls from within, techniques for the treatment of the aggressive child*. New York, NY: Free Press/Macmillan.

Smith, A. (1977). An inquiry into the nature and causes of *The Wealth of Nations*. Edwin Cannan (Ed.). New York, NY: The Modern Library. (Original work published 1776)

CHAPTER THREE

THE INITIAL TREATMENT PLAN

*I*nitial treatment planning in the partial hospitalization program (PHP)/ intensive outpatient program (IOP) setting is not merely used to create a document but is both the road map and the pacesetter for the patient's expected progress. With some exceptions,[1] it is

- The beginning of the relationship with the patient and the family that can set the tone for treatment
- The entry of the patient into the milieu that can lead to a patient's positive role in the milieu
- The baseline by which to measure progress
- The rationale for continued treatment and reimbursement for services

Initial treatment planning can be a challenging if not frustrating endeavor with all that is expected of the PHP/IOP clinician. Treatment planning does not happen by itself, but is one of the myriad tasks that a clinician must perform under deadlines and in the intense PHP/IOP milieu.

Conceiving initial treatment planning as a game is a helpful framework for organizing and executing this task in the intense PHP/IOP setting; this chapter lays out how to play it. It reviews the limits the clinician faces in conducting treatment planning as a game. It also discusses reasonable expectations in goal constructing. It suggests a game consisting of scripts and methods for treatment planning.

---

[1] Exceptions include the program design in which the patient is in group sessions before meeting for individual treatment planning, how savvy the patient in treatment is, whether the patient is a returning patient, and whether the patient is a personality-disordered individual.

THE ESSENCE OF TREATMENT PLANNING

Inherently, when it comes to treatment planning, each problem suggests the goals, strategies, and tasks that lead to the patient's progress. Each patient's baseline functioning level suggests some strategies. Furthermore, given the nature of PHP/IOP, the strategies usually consist of a solution set: (a) psychopharmacology/medication, (b) participation in group therapy, and (c) independent goals the patient pursues that will further his or her recovery. A family member or close supportive person may be involved in creating and fulfilling the goals. If family therapy is part of the treatment plan, how the family sessions go has an impact on patient progress. In theory, the combination of the strategies and tasks used help the patient benefit from the PHP/IOP treatment.

In line with the economy view of the milieu discussed in Chapter 2, initial treatment planning is an economic good that the clinician offers. The clinician makes a connection with the patient, and when necessary, with the patient's family, to connect the problems with the paths to recovery. The quality of initial treatment planning is based on how the clinician (a) efficiently joins and attends[2] with the patient and family, (b) offers hope, and (c) gives information as to how recovery theoretically progresses. Both the poise and professional stance of the clinician are crucial in initial treatment planning.

The hallmark of professional poise and stance is *active listening* and *attending* with *direct eye contact* and a *soft but firm tone of voice*. Simply being able to repeat to the patient what the patient said has surprising effectiveness for the PHP/IOP patient in distress.[3] Otherwise, program staff can look incompetent when a patient does not express the satisfaction that he or she has been heard and understood.[4] Patients and their

---

[2] *Joining* is defined here as beginning a relationship with the patient and the family. *Attending* is defined here as empathetically responding to the emotional and informational expression of the patient and the family.

[3] In a sense, this does borrow from the Milton Erickson school of thought. Repetition of the patient's own words can be even more effective. However, sometimes the clinician may have to explore the significance of the *depression* or *anxiety* to the patient.

[4] Often, there are clinicians who, out of their personal anxieties, do not trust the intake assessments and want to make their own assessment from scratch. Some agencies/hospitals exude incompetence when clinicians do not trust the information passed on from admission or intake.

families can express irritation and annoyance when they have to recite problems over and over again to a new clinician.

Even though it can reflect on the clinician, the biggest roadblock to treatment success is the patient's failure to demonstrate responsibility. Patients come to the program with different levels of acuity and cognitive functioning, and thus with different sets of abilities and inabilities. Many patients and their families also come with agendas of avoidance or escape and are covert in their actual reasons for seeking treatment; their solutions to their problems are being in the program and not necessarily addressing psychiatric symptoms through the PHP/IOP. A patient who is unmotivated or incapable will demonstrate poor compliance and likely have minimal progress.[5]

THE LIMITS OF INITIAL TREATMENT PLANNING

Besides the dependence on the patient's motivation, treatment planning in PHP/IOP is constrained by time limits, insurance/funding limits, the program design limits, the treatment cohort, and census size. Understanding and appreciating these limits is crucial to successfully playing this game.

The first limit is time. The average PHP/IOP clinician has multiple tasks and multiple deadlines. The typical PHP/IOP clinician is stretched in multiple directions and has limited time with each patient to be thorough and to formulate effective goals.

Second, since the PHP/IOP has parameters, the treatment plan can address only the salient functioning issues before the patient is discharged.[6] Given the utilization or insurance standards for PHP/IOP care,

---

[5] Many treatment-savvy patients are examples of unmotivated patients. They know how treatment works and are dismissive of feedback from a clinician, but they do not appear to demonstrate or relate that they are responsible for their own recovery.

[6] An adolescent patient who reports transgender identity issues as a stressor is unlikely to have this issue resolved. Issues such as anxiety and depression may be more reasonable to address in this situation. More information on this matter can be found from the Henry Benjamin standards of care: http://www.wpath .org/documents2/socv6.pdf

if a patient has improved to a certain level and is no longer showing certain symptoms, he or she will no longer meet the criteria required to stay in the program.

Third, a treatment plan is limited by the cognitive abilities or agenda of the patient and the family. The anxious adult patient often has unrealistic desires to solve all the problems that led to admission. A significantly depressed or anxious patient is unlikely to have full cognitive abilities for truly identifying treatment needs.[7] The patient stepping down from inpatient care may not be able to identify the reason for admission other than psychiatrist referral.[8] Furthermore, the patient who is embarrassed, ashamed, or guarded about the reasons for admission may not give the salient details to a stranger (in this case, a clinician), and the goals may not be relevant or valid because the patient has withheld information.[9] Another challenge is the oppositional adolescent or child who denies a need for treatment. Although the list can go on, a patient and family can be lower functioning, resistant to change, and in perpetual drama, all of which hamper the creation of a realistic treatment plan. Therefore a treatment plan will only be as valid as the truthfulness and ability of the patient.

Fourth, another treatment plan limitation goes a little further when dealing with a child or adolescent patient and his or her family. Family secrets and dysfunction come into play. In family systems, the child is often the identified patient who reflects larger issues. Parents may be problem focused, may only focus on the child's behavior, and may not want to talk about goals. Parents often deny that they contribute to the

---

[7] Someone in a depressed episode of bipolar disorder is generally a poor historian and has distorted thinking about what is normal. For this type of patient, the manic episode is considered to be normal or desired.

[8] Even though they are not fully recovered, depressed adult patients stepping down from inpatient care may state that they do not have any problems and do not have any particular goals to work on. The patients may say that the psychiatrist recommended admission. Such patients are likely at the beginning hump of the recovery process (see Figure 1.2 in Chapter 1).

[9] Someone with a personality disorder or personality-disorder traits tends to have a distorted view of the facts and is considered to lack insight into his or her responsibility for the situation. Some patients may also be using treatment to avoid work or delay employee discipline and job termination.

problem and view the child's behavior as the sole problem.[10] Some parents project their own emotions onto their children in claiming the child has anger issues, when the child is reacting to the parent's dysfunctional or abusive behavior. Furthermore, the parent(s) and the patient may be in "the wrong," against the system but may deny they are doing anything wrong.[11] Thus, in child/adolescent situations, it often helps to look at the initial treatment plans as being preliminary, because more information may be disclosed later.

Fifth, the average program has a design intended for a specific treatment cohort. The program must use strategies consisting of the treatment modalities in the program design. Goals must fit how the patient can use the modalities. The patient must be able to participate in the program in both physical and cognitive terms.[12]

Sixth, treatment plans in the PHP/IOP setting are time limited and behavioral in nature. The treatment plan measures the patient's behavioral health or demonstrated behaviors over an allowable period of time. If the patient does not demonstrate the behaviors specified by the treatment plan (to be extinguished and/or reinforced), the payer source may not approve more visits if the patient does not have severe symptomology.[13] If a patient says "I want to feel better" and cannot verbalize what "feeling better" means, then the clinician may have to discuss behavioral

---

[10] In a case in which the child/adolescent patient has observable depressive or psychotic symptoms, a psychosocial or systems analysis has less importance than psychopharmacology and resolving symptoms.

[11] In cases in which child protective services/child welfare is involved, and the family is highly enmeshed, the family may defocus and go off on multiple tangents.

[12] Many programs say that they will serve anyone, but in practical terms, they do not budget for additional services to serve those with special needs. Generally, the patient's needs must be met within the time frames of the program. If the patient has special needs that require care that takes longer than the breaks, and the patient is missing group sessions, then the patient is unable to benefit from the designed program modalities. The patient must also meet a certain amount of intellectual functioning for certain types of insight-based interventions.

[13] This can be both in terms of the adult who is to show behavioral improvement in anxiety, depression, and psychotic symptoms and in terms of the child/adolescent with oppositional and anger management issues.

examples of "feeling better" and suggest options.[14] If a patient wants to fix every problem, the clinician will have to educate the patient on what is reasonable.

In line with the patient's "problems," the clinician may have to shape the goals or reframe for the patient what is reasonable within the available time limits. Some patients say that "other people" are the problem. Although the other people in the patient's life may be difficult or problematic, what the patient is going to choose to do with that situation is a more reasonable treatment focus. In such a case, the clinician may need to suggest goals such as "The patient will talk in group therapy about family relationships."[15]

A different limitation is presented by the clinician. The clinician may be inexperienced for a particular situation and face a learning curve. On the other hand, the clinician may realize the feeling of countertransference, in which it may not be in either the patient's interest or the clinician's interest for a relationship to continue. When a PHP/IOP clinician realizes that a case is beyond his or her skills or experience, the clinician should get supervision or case consultation or review it as soon as possible with the psychiatrist or an available doctor.

The clinician's workload bears mentioning, as the clinician is essentially a detail-oriented multitasker in this setting, who seeks to maximize efficiencies while being as effective as possible. Having more patients means more work for the clinician in a limited amount of time. Treatment planning is a challenge in terms of the clinician's efficiency and effectiveness. Therefore, trying to get the patient's whole story is often unnecessary and inefficient in this setting. There are problems and then there are treatment priorities. Not all problems must be addressed, nor can they be addressed in treatment. Some patients supply a lengthy list of problems that can clutter a treatment plan. Some patients given to drama and codependency may be focused on the problems of others that are outside of their responsibility and control. The efficient and effective clinician

---

[14] The Joint Commission, which is the de facto accreditation organization in the United States, has made it a standard that the goals be in the patient's words.

[15] In this case, the assumption is that the therapy group will give rational feedback to the patient about the inability to change family members and help the patient identify some coping skills.

therefore serves as a guide for the patient as to what the reasonable and appropriate expectations in the PHP/IOP are.

REASONABLE EXPECTATIONS

Reasonable (as a term in the case of treatment planning) means moderate or not excessive (*Merriam-Webster's Collegiate Dictionary*, 2005). A reasonable treatment plan means that the goals are likely to be achieved within the time limits that the pertinent managed care organization allows, and rarely is the patient going to fix "all" of the problems.

Reasonable also means that the goals are appropriate[16] for the patient's problem(s), available resources, and the patient's functioning level. Being reasonable may include accepting that the patient is going to resolve just the essential problems in order to return to regular functioning.

The functioning level with which the patient presents is the starting point for considering what is reasonable. With many patients, the goals should move from the simple to the more complex. Scenarios of reasonable expectations include the following:

- A severely depressed patient with high levels of anxiety is unlikely to engage in cognitive behavioral therapy strategies until the medication starts working to enable the patient to process and retain information. *(The patient should attend group therapy and talk when prompted and demonstrate completion of activities of daily living [ADLs].)*
- An agoraphobic patient may have to start being compliant in attending the program and practicing basic coping skills before going back to work. *(The patient should attend every day and talk about anxiety.)*
- A child with attention deficit hyperactivity disorder (ADHD), anger management, and school problems must take medication consistently and be monitored in the program before the child can learn coping skills. *(The child should attend every day and take the prescribed medication.)*
- The suicidal patient should focus on goals of maintaining personal safety versus the goal of trying to get back to work. *(The patient will cooperate in the removal of all weapons or other means of suicide.)*

---

[16] *Appropriate* does not have to connote *precision* and can mean a range of possible options.

Although some psychiatrists are conservative with medication and focus on therapy and coping skills, the typical PHP/IOP patient should have a goal to be compliant with medication as prescribed.

GOALS

Besides the matter of medication compliance, identifying goals to be used in a PHP/IOP setting may be a matter of politics. Much of what is used for goals depends on preexisting rights and the products purchased by organizations. Many hospitals have software packages that integrate goals, documentation, and billing that have prescribed sets of goals. Utilization review standards such as InterQual[17] or the managed care organizations themselves can dictate patient goals.

Some general examples of initial goals include the following:

- The patient will evidence no further self-harm.
- The patient will abstain from the use of alcohol and/or substances.
- The patient will engage in mood-stabilizing behavior, including _____.
- The patient will participate in program activities.
- The patient will identify ___ coping skills.
- The patient will identify ___ illness signs and symptoms.
- The patient will demonstrate stabilization as evidenced by _____.
- The patient will identify ___ (anxiety, anger, or relapse) triggers.
- The patient will do the following homework: _____.
- The patient will demonstrate medication compliance.
- The patient will attend ____ self-help meetings.
- The family and patient will meet for ___ sessions for the purpose of _____.
- The patient will talk in group therapy about his or her feelings and situation.
- The patient will demonstrate completion of ADLs.

Any of these goals can include specific (or concrete) elaborations of the expected behavioral outcome. The coping skills goal can be applied to

---

[17] InterQual is a utilization management standard that is published by the McKesson Corporation (Mitus, 2008).

anxiety, depression, suicidal ideation, or even anger. The trigger identification goals can be applied to self-harm, trauma, eating disorders, or relapse. Regardless of the goal selection in initial treatment planning, simple is better. Hopefully, the patient can identify desired goals. Goals indicate that the patient desires to get better and is motivated to participate in the treatment.

THE PROCESS OF GETTING STARTED

The clinician has four inherent tasks in initial treatment planning: (a) to quantify the patient's acuity, (b) to make sure the patient is safe and not a danger to self or others, (c) to get the patient/family to agree to a set of treatment goals that will address the problems, and (d) to get the patient's commitment to stay in treatment. The first task is relatively easy; the second task is not guaranteed. The hurdle to getting this started is "joining" (Minuchin, 1974) with the family. In the joining process, the clinician is entering into the world of the patient and the family to gain trust, understand the problem, and identify what to do about it.

Joining with the patient and/or the family will vary with the situation. Much of how the clinician joins with the patient and/or family depends on whether there is advance notice and on how much time the clinician has to review admission and inpatient documents. On the flip side, the clinician may have some hurdle with an acutely symptomatic patient who is labile, psychotic, guarded, paranoid, or acting entitled. When the clinician has little to no advance notice of a new patient and does not get the admission documents, he or she will need to depend on a patient interview. The patient may want to rush out as soon as possible and hopefully will have completed enough of an admission survey. Keeping the four tasks in mind helps the clinician develop flexibility with the different patient scenarios.

In adult settings, the patient will likely come alone to the initial treatment planning session. In child and adolescent settings, the clinician will meet the patient with the guardian, parent(s), or family. In geriatric settings, the family may also be present at initial treatment planning. Joining with the family and the patient together may make the situation more complex than when the patient is alone.

Every new patient encounter is a calculated risk, as there are multiple dynamics in the initial treatment planning session that can impact the joining process and impede initial treatment planning. The risk includes the patient and/or family member(s) showing transference toward the clinician or the clinician showing countertransference toward the patient. The patient with higher levels of anxiety or mood lability seen in a PHP/IOP setting more likely will show transference.[18] A patient who has significant trauma or neglect history may demonstrate reluctance or guardedness in discussing problems and goals. When a family is involved, the therapist can be thrown into a drama as a persecutor or villain in the process of exploring goals.[19] The clinician can also encounter a guarded patient and/or family who see the clinician as part of a distrusted system as a result of the family's previous interaction with child welfare/child protection agencies. In a grand sense, these patient and/or family situations are examples of challenges to joining with the family.

The general answer to dealing with multiple dynamics, whether transference, family dysfunction, or symbolic distrust, is the development of a general set of standards that include the clinician not acting in a defensive manner but maintaining a calm and mature posture and tone. The clinician's adherence to standards implies that this relationship and encounter are not personal but objective, professional, and factual. When they become personal, it means the clinician has lost objectivity.

However, out of fear and defensiveness, many patients and families will engage in personalization[20] with the clinician. They may defensively scapegoat professionals as the symbolic face of the system. They may project emotion on the clinician. They may say that they do not like the clinician. They may immediately request another clinician.[21] Stepping back and empathetically acknowledging that the patients and their families

---

[18] This patient may have personality-disorder traits.

[19] The scenario of the adolescent or child who has truancy issues of not wanting to start the program the day of admission indicates enmeshment between the parent and child. The personality-disordered parent will put forth some kind of victim status in stating that he or she is helpless. Sometimes there are family secrets that the family is trying to protect at the onset and so the first clinician is a sacrificial lamb.

[20] In cognitive-behavioral thought, personalization is a cognitive distortion in which a matter is irrationally made personal or taken personally.

[21] Personality-disordered or controlling patients, and their parents, often "fire" the first clinician. This is a way of maintaining distance and controlling the situation.

have negative feelings about the system may improve the compliance of the patient and the family in getting the initial treatment plan completed.

Actually Starting: The Script

Given all of the limitations and challenges of creating a treatment plan, the best strategy to use in initial treatment planning is using a script. In its essential form, a script is both the information to be communicated and the manner of presentation or delivery. The material is readily identifiable, but the manner of delivery is complicated with many potential nuances. The script is therefore more than its words and nuances; it is a structured plan.

The strategy of the treatment planning script is to identify the patient's relevant past, relevant present, and desired future. Although the anxious patient may report a lot of information, relatively little of this can be addressed by the clinician and the program. The script of initial treatment planning must identify:

- The patient's crucial issues that led to admission
- The patient's priorities
- The patient's current functioning problems
- The patient's current clinical measurements (often called "clinicals")
- The patient's goals, wishes, or desires

Script nuances can include tone of voice, facial expression, and attitude.[22] In conjunction with the general set of standards for the clinician, these nuances indicate that the prescribed clinician presentation is that of a mature adult in control of his or her emotions. The clinician's tone of voice and facial expression should not be theatrical, but confident and calm.

The script includes spelling out for the patient and the family the objective of the meeting. In the case of initial treatment planning in the PHP/IOP setting, the script should be directive. It should include the following elements:

- The intended meeting time limit
- The purpose

---

[22] *Attitude* here refers to thought content and the emotions that go with it.

- Reasons for admission
- Review of progress
- Current mental status or state
- Goals to be achieved
- Discharge plan
- Any other essential information that the patient deems important

A script that is directive and open helps give the anxious or paranoid patient a message that the conference is to be a straightforward encounter. A useful script that has been in use for some time is Studer Group's AIDET®, which stands for:

- Acknowledge
- Introduce
- Duration
- Explanation
- Thank You[23]

Sometimes, there is just not enough time for an adequate or thorough interview to develop an effective, initial treatment plan. The use of an intake survey can be helpful for a number of cohorts. An example of such a survey is found in Appendix A.

When a survey is not used, or the patient refuses/is unable to complete a survey, having a copy of the admission/intake assessment is essential. Although the patient's perspective and information may change from the date of the admitting assessment, it can be the starting point of the script.

A program's capacity and funding source inherently influences the type of script the clinician uses. Although building space and management philosophies can dictate how large a PHP/IOP will grow, in the United States, Medicaid and Medicare rules inherently limit therapy

---

[23] Studer Group is the originator of the AIDET method. Studer Group has published AIDET in multiple materials, including through its publishing arm, Fire Starter Publishing. The organization does not cite one seminal work for this concept. One specific work in which the reader can find out more about this is: Studer Group. (n.d.) *AIDET® five fundamentals of patient communication* (DVD). Gulf Breeze, FL: Fire Starter Publishing.

group sizes. If the program has a limited capacity, admissions are scheduled and a clinician likely has a more regulated work schedule with advance notice and access to the admission/intake assessment. Commercial insurance has no capacity limit, so in these cases, the clinician may have little to no advance notice of a new admission and may need to use an intake survey as part of the script in order to get all the necessary tasks completed.[24]

The Opening Script

The following is an example of an opening script based on AIDET used when the clinician has possession of the intake/admitting assessment:

> Hello, I'm Dave. I'm a social worker here, and I will be doing the admission. I got advance notice of your coming, and I reviewed the problems and needs that brought you here. In the next 15 minutes, I want to make sure I understand what happened, how things have improved, what we need to do, and get the necessary papers signed.

The following is an example of an opening script used when the clinician has no advance notice:

> Hi, my name is Dave. I'm a social worker here and I will be doing your admission. My goals in the next 15 minutes are to understand what brought you here, what we need to accomplish, and where we need to go when you're done. Then we will sign the necessary papers.

A third example of an opening script is a matter-of-fact script used when the clinician is pressed for time and there has been no advance notice.

> Hi, I'm Dave. I am going to be your social worker. I need to be honest with you in that I am crunched for time right now. I'm sorry for that. Maybe we can meet later or tomorrow to talk more if you need to. I want to avoid having you repeat the whole story that brought you here, but I need to understand the main reasons you need to be here and what we most need to do for you.

---

[24] The presence of even one Medicaid or Medicare patient in a therapy group in the United States requires the group to be capitated or limited in size.

With this third example, the clinician's tone must be soft, calm, warm, but direct. The clinician's apology is sincere because the patient is indeed a valuable person and the reason that the clinician is there and getting paid. The impression the clinician is trying to make is that this is not personal, but a condition of the situation. An arrogant clinician may alienate and lose clients.

The opening script implies an open door between the clinician and patient. Although the clinician is politely setting limits as part of the milieu, he or she is aiming to be in a position to receive new and crucial clinical information as it comes.

The Middle Interview

The middle part of the interview script is the clinical information that is needed to justify the patient's reason for being in the program and ensuring the patient's safety. This information is collected either through the survey or through direct interviewing of the patient. This clinical information includes mental status, mood, anxiety, and functioning.[25]

Mental status requirements are objective pieces of information that the clinician can gather by observing the patient. But in the end, they are dependent on the subjective view of the patient. What a program or clinician chooses to ask is for the most part arbitrary, but common elements are:

- Time (What day is it?)
- Place (Where are you?)
- Person (Who are you?)
- Appearance (How is the patient's hygiene and appearance?)
- Thought content (How is the patient thinking? Logically? Concretely? Problems completing thoughts?)
- Affect (What mood does the patient appear to have?)
- Hallucinations (Does the patient report hearing voices or seeing things?)[26]

---

[25] Some payer sources may require additional mental status information such as a formal Mini–Mental State Examination.

[26] Hallucinations can be auditory, visual, olfactory (smell), and tactile (feeling).

- Delusions (Does the patient report paranoia or show delusional thinking?)[27]
- Suicidal ideation (Is the patient having any thoughts of suicide?)
- Homicidal ideation (Is the patient having any thoughts of hurting someone?)

Sometimes the patient may need reassessment for inpatient admission depending on the answers supplied in the interview, as acuity can actually get worse between the initial assessment and actual admission to the PHP/IOP.[28]

DEPRESSION AND ANXIETY SCALES

Depression and anxiety are subjective emotional states. Although there are objectively observable symptoms that indicate their presence, they remain subjective concepts. The clinician can make an objective observation about the patient's mood and anxiety, but merely communicating to an insurance reviewer how the patient looked may not get any more coverage or further approval. What is often expected is a report of the patient's depression and anxiety in terms of a numerical score that communicates the degree of severity.[29]

A numerical score for depression and anxiety typically follows a 0 to 5 or a 0 to 10 scale. Here, "0" usually means the least or lowest score, whereas "10" is the highest score, with all numbers in between suggesting some moderation.

---

[27] Delusions are more likely to be of a paranoid type in which the patient is worried that people are watching him or her. If a patient has significant paranoia, the patient will likely express the paranoia, which may include that the government is bugging the house or that everyone is watching him or her. One common delusion is that others are out to poison the patient.

[28] This can happen as a patient may just be "on the line" at initial assessment and can worsen in the time between assessment and admission. The patient may also disclose more at admission than he or she did at assessment.

[29] In essence, the clinician is converting a nominal variable (all there or all not there) into an ordinal variable indicating some rank order. Considering depression and anxiety scales as interval or continuous variables presents both validity and reliability risks.

0	1–2	3–4	5–6	7–8	9–10
Content, not depressed	Down, mild depression	Sad, moderate depression	Blue, severe depression	Unhappy, very severe depression	Hopeless, suicidal, worst depression
0	1–2	3–4	5–6	7–8	9–10
Calm, content, not anxious	Concerned, tense, mild anxiety	Worried, moderate anxiety	Jumpy/edgy, severe anxiety	Fearful, very severe anxiety	Panic attacks/pain, worst anxiety

Figure 3.1[30] *Sample mood and anxiety scales.*

Using only numbers can be acceptable, but there is the risk of vagueness and misunderstanding.[31] The numbers can mean whatever the patient wants them to mean, which can be different from the clinician's view. Furthermore, the use of a numbers-only scale can invite distortion when patients want to give themselves a 22 on a scale of 10.

The scale should be simple and easy to understand. Using numbers and words in the scale cues the patient on what is appropriate and provides mutual understanding of the patient's anxiety and depression levels. Figure 3.1 provides suggested mood and anxiety scales for use in PHP/IOP.

The mood and anxiety scales can be used in a patient admission survey or as a chart to which the clinician refers the patient in the course of the interview. The clinician has some flexibility in using the scales with patients depending on time limits, patient cognitive functioning, and even budgetary issues.

FUNCTIONING

As discussed in Chapter 1, the patient's level of functioning is a determinant of the level of care where a patient will be placed. Assuming that the patient already has had an initial assessment in the hospital/organization admitting department, the functioning information may already be

---

[30] Thanks to Michael Taylor, LMFT, for this configuration.

[31] A very depressed patient may not have the cognitive ability to make a determination solely based on a numerical scale.

in that document. At the risk of repetition, the clinician can ask a number of questions that include the following:

- When were you last at work or school?
- How are you at doing your ADLs (bathing, grooming, and changing clothes)?
- What kinds of activities have you not been able to do lately?
- How have you been sleeping?
- How is your appetite?
- Have you been drinking alcohol or using street drugs?[32] If so, how much?

Some of the functioning responses can be shaped into goals. For example, if the patient's hygiene is observed to be a functioning problem—and admitted by the patient to be a problem—then a relevant and reasonable treatment goal could be added that the patient will demonstrate success with a regimen of daily hygiene.

THE FINAL PART OF THE INTERVIEW

Regardless of the approach, when the interview appears to be closing, there are a number of patient questions that allow for efficiency, thoroughness, and risk reduction:

- Do I have things correct?
- Are there any other facts I am missing or need to understand?
- Is there anything else I need to know that I have not asked about?

There is the risk that the depressed and anxious/scared patient (who may have never had counseling or therapy) goes along with the clinician's agenda and withholds information because the clinician does not specifically ask for it. These disclosures can include the following:

---

[32] This assumes that the patient has been sent to the program for psychiatric problems and not chemical dependency problems. There are many patients who present as coming for psychiatric treatment who do not disclose their alcohol and/or substance use.

- The patient is a victim of domestic violence.
- The patient discloses suicidal thoughts not reported at assessment.
- The patient is a victim of rape.
- The patient committed a crime.
- The patient has a sexual issue.[33]

If the patient adds information that suggests a new problem, the clinician can determine with the patient whether the new information needs to be part of the treatment focus.[34]

On the other hand, an important "economic" value of the interview is that the patient agrees that he or she was heard and was understood. Even though the clinician is often in a hurry and has a sizeable workload, the impression that the clinician thoroughly and empathetically heard the patient goes far in keeping a patient coming to a program.

DETERMINING SUCCESS IN THE GAME OF INITIAL TREATMENT PLANNING

In keeping with the concept of the game, the standard of clinician success in the game of initial treatment planning is that within all the limits and challenges of the situation, the following tasks are completed:

- The clinician has guided the patient in selecting/agreeing to reasonable goals.
- The goals are likely achievable during the time the patient attends the program.
- The clinician has the necessary clinical information for utilization review.

---

[33] Sometimes, the additional issue is not reported in the admission statement due to patient reluctance or embarrassment. This is an opportunity for the clinician to show acceptance of the patient and quickly build an alliance.

[34] As stated earlier, not all problems that the patient mentions can be the focus of treatment in the PHP/IOP setting. This can be due either to the nature of the patient's stated problem or to the length of time the patient is going to be in the program. Sometimes, the new problem does not require immediate attention.

- The clinician is able to complete the documentation within the deadlines.
- The patient returns the next day for treatment.

In playing the game, it is up to each clinician to decide on a style that works for the clinician. There are numerous ways to play the game of treatment planning well. A PHP/IOP clinician should regularly evaluate, experiment, and polish treatment planning activities. When polished and done well, initial treatment planning leads to increased efficiency, effectiveness, and patient satisfaction.

CONCLUSIONS

This chapter discussed the game of initial treatment planning, which is the creation of a road map and pacesetting for a patient's expected progress. Initial treatment planning is crucial in terms of identifying the patient's acuity level, identifying expected treatment progress, and securing reimbursement for the PHP/IOP services.

With all of its challenges and limits, treatment planning is where the PHP/IOP clinician is expected to bring order amid chaos. The clinician aims to provide the patient and the family a sense of hope that the problems that brought the patient to the program can be treated and that the patient will improve. Within a limited period of time, the clinician politely and professionally elicits a lot of clinical information from the patient and the family and shapes it into goals and usable information that will secure reimbursement from payer sources. The clinician also has to guide and educate the patient and the family about reasonable expectations and goals. The PHP/IOP clinician must do initial treatment planning in the midst of numerous other clinical tasks.

This chapter proposed the development and use of a script. In its most basic form, the script is an organized plan. The script can be simple or complex.

The PHP/IOP clinician's script includes not only the introduction and the questions needed to gather the information but also addresses the clinician's tone and attitude. The clinician's tone and attitude should be those of a mature adult in control. The clinician attends to the patient's/family member's emotions; he or she does not react when the patient or family member lashes out but stays in control of emotion and maintains a professional perspective. This paraverbal aspect is crucial in maintaining focus on achieving the task of treatment planning in a reasonable amount of time and not getting distracted by family or patient drama.

The clinician should develop several treatment planning scripts for the recurring scenarios in the program. Typically, there are two or three scenarios that reflect the opportunity, or lack of it, to prepare and the time limitations imposed. Developing the script as the strategy for successful initial treatment planning is a learning process. At first, any script can be wooden, but with practice and refinement, it is an effective tool. Part of a clinician's success in the game is practicing and refining the script so that more competent clinical work is done in less time.

REFERENCES

Merriam-Webster's collegiate dictionary (11th ed.). (2005). Springfield, MA: Merriam-Webster.

Minuchin, S. (1974). *Families & family therapy.* Cambridge, MA: Harvard University Press.

Mitus, A. J. (2008). The birth of InterQual: Evidence-based decision support criteria that helped change healthcare. *Professional Case Management, 13,* 228–233.

CHAPTER FOUR

CONCURRENT TREATMENT PLANNING

Concurrent treatment planning is the process of measuring progress, identifying further patient goals, and clarifying when the patient is ready for discharge. Concurrent treatment planning often takes place in the context of tension between what the patient wants to happen, what the clinician observes to be happening, and what a managed care reviewer (or care manager) expects to be happening.

Concurrent treatment planning is built on the initial treatment plan and any events[1] that happened since admission. This chapter is written under the assumption that the clinician is dealing with managed care[2] in which concurrent treatment planning is conducted at set intervals or at the will of the managed care organization (MCO).[3] When concurrent treatment planning is at the will of the MCO, the clinician is challenged to articulate a patient's acuity and a rationale for additional patient-days.[4] In the absence of such MCO demand, concurrent review is conducted at

---

[1] Events refer to therapy progress, failure to progress, or other events in the life of the patient.

[2] Berger (2002) gives a brief history of managed care's genesis in the United States. He also characterizes utilization review as a cost-control strategy of managed care. His two categories of control include utilization controls and reimbursement and payment controls. Concurrent review is one of the utilization controls (Berger, 2002). MacKenzie (1995) observes that managed care has been a trend in Western countries (pp. 1–4).

[3] The MCO can be the insurer itself, a contractor of the insurance company, or a subcontractor of the contractor. An MCO is typically a for-profit company incentivized to make money by saving money. Money that does not get spent on service fees goes to the MCO's bottom line.

[4] A patient-day is a unit of measurement in health care that refers to 1 day of care given to one patient.

standard intervals in accordance with accreditation or government standards or a psychiatrist's preference.[5]

This chapter is written with another assumption: that the clinician is responsible for treatment planning in the PHP/IOP setting. In some programs, nurses are responsible for treatment planning and may consult the clinician for input.[6]

This chapter explores the game of concurrent treatment planning in the PHP/IOP setting, where the clinician has the responsibility for identifying a patient's treatment progress and documenting the patient's continued acuity to get more covered days from MCOs. It discusses utilization management and its role in treatment planning. It discusses the challenges and tasks of concurrent treatment planning. A game plan is suggested for getting the right information for follow-up treatment planning. The game of concurrent treatment planning includes cooperating with utilization reviews or utilization departments to get additional covered patient-days and handling the dreaded peer-to-peer review.

THE BASICS OF UTILIZATION REVIEW

Utilization review is a process that determines whether a patient needs further treatment or should be discharged.[7] The determination is made based on criteria established in the contract between the insurance carrier and the provider. The criteria are typically organized in a decision-tree format that the payer source follows in making payment decisions. As part of the contract, the payer source or MCO makes the criteria available to the hospital or agency.

---

[5] Some organizations have a protocol of the psychiatrist leading a treatment team. In the absence of a protocol, involvement level is based on the preference of the psychiatrist.

[6] Ideally, this will be a collaborative process that includes clinician input. The reviewer may call the clinician for input if the resulting treatment plan is deemed to be inadequate.

[7] In the United States, MCOs control the criteria for treatment, the number of days they will certify, and the frequency of review. They save money by giving fewer days and requiring frequent review-scrutinizing details of a patient's demonstrated symptomology and functioning.

The criteria for continued care vary according to the payer source or MCO[8] and how the contract was written. The criteria are usually categorized according to clinical problem areas[9] and are purported to be evidence based, with multiple bibliographic citations referring to research. The utilization review criteria dictate that certain services be provided to the patient within certain time frames or benchmarks. The reviewer looks at the clinical documentation of the patient progress and symptomology at the time of the review. Either the patient does or does not meet the criteria for admission (if initial review) or continued treatment (if concurrent review).

The clinician and/or physician bear the weight of proof in utilization reviews for authorized days in treatment. On admission, the admitting clinician typically calls the MCO or insurance company and states the clinical justification for treatment. If the MCO or insurance reviewer agrees that the patient meets the criteria for the designated level of care, then the patient will be authorized a limited number of days of treatment. If the MCO reviewer does not authorize the treatment, the case is either denied or it is sent for a *doc-to-doc* or *peer-to-peer* review in which either the clinician or the psychiatrist must review with the MCO's contracted or employed physician to justify the admission.

If the MCO denies the admission, the organization may admit the patient and appeal the denial. If the patient is admitted and then denied more days at the time of a concurrent review, the patient is often kept in the hospital, based on the hospital policy and physician opinion.[10] Often, the hospital will appeal the denial to the MCO in hopes that the additional patient information will suffice to get reimbursement for the services.

---

[8] The MCOs vary in modus operandi and utilization criteria. The utilization criteria are often considered to be "proprietary" information, which is not readily shared with providers. MCOs may require immediate review on admission and approve fewer or more days at a time. The behavior of an MCO also depends on an individual reviewer's arbitrary preferences or behaviors.

[9] Problem areas usually are mood, anxiety, mania, psychosis, substance use, and disruptive behavior.

[10] In U.S. cases of commercial insurance denial, a patient is often given an option of paying the cash rate if the patient wants to stay in treatment.

If the MCO authorizes the admission, it will certify a specific number of covered[11] days before the next review and expect a number of specified services be delivered to the patient and documented in the medical record by the time of the next review. The services can include daily clinical assessment, psychiatric assessment, and attendance in programming for a minimum number of hours per day over a specified number of days. The MCO may dictate the delivery of additional services for a continued patient stay. Some of the services may include a mental status examination, substance abuse evaluation, or a family session. A managed care reviewer may seek information of questionable relevance and dictate obtuse actions, but because of the managed care reviewer's position of power, the clinician will need to comply and provide answers.[12] The MCO will expect a report on the outcomes at the next review, and if the directives are not followed or are not delivered, the MCO may not authorize any more covered days.

Some MCOs dictate at admission a limited number of days and expect discharge to regular outpatient care. If the patient is a "step-down" from inpatient, the MCO may have made this statement when the patient was still hospitalized. Hopefully, this limit is communicated to the clinician at admission, and the clinician can join with the patient quickly to create a treatment plan in accordance with a time frame dictated by the MCO reviewer.

The MCO will usually give an expiration date for the number of certified patient-days. In these cases, the MCO will expect the certified days to be used by that expiration date and will not allow any missed days to be used after that date unless there is an acceptable explanation.[13]

---

[11] *Covered* refers to the MCO's agreement to pay for the services. However, the MCO gives a usual disclaimer that authorization is not a guarantee of payment.

[12] Within their own organizational parameters, MCO reviewers do have the power to approve additional days. MCO reviewers may insist that protective welfare services be called in situations for which the clinician does not see a need for such reporting.

[13] The acceptable explanation needs to be a crisis of a medical or family nature. Otherwise, being in a PHP or IOP is a priority. The assumption is that if the patient is not attending the program, he or she is not in need of the services.

The typical clinician in a hospital will have a utilization review department staffed by nurses or other clinicians who communicate with the MCO. These utilization reviewers are usually exclusive liaisons between the program or physician and the insurance companies or MCOs.[14] Nevertheless, the in-house utilization reviewer will review the patient's chart for symptomology and progress even when the patient's payer source is not an MCO.

After chart review, a utilization reviewer will contact the clinician for clarifying information on a patient. Such clarification is used to determine the patient's needs and to communicate the terms of the MCO authorization. The utilization reviewer may report that there is inadequate support for a continued patient stay and request more clinical information. When there is inadequate evidence for a continued stay, the clinician bears the onus of gathering the necessary information and reporting back to the utilization reviewer.

The utilization reviewer will relate the patient's clinical information to the MCO reviewer. If the MCO reviewer agrees that more treatment is indicated, he or she will grant certification for more days. If the MCO reviewer does not agree that more treatment is needed, more coverage is denied or the case is sent for peer-to-peer or doc-to-doc review.[15]

The peer-to-peer review is an exercise of greater MCO scrutiny of whether or not a patient meets the criteria for care. Some MCOs have protocols as to when a case is to go peer to peer. A case can go for a peer-to-peer review when:

- The MCO care manager does feel there is enough evidence for an admission or a continued stay.
- The MCO decision tree indicates a case is to go for a peer-to-peer review.
- The patient continues to have persistent symptomology and more days of coverage are asked for by the clinician.

---

[14] Solo clinicians running their own IOPs do their own utilization reviews and talk directly to the insurance companies or MCOs.

[15] *Peer to peer* is the choice of term in this chapter. *Doc to doc* is also used; this is when the psychiatrist reviews the case with an MCO doctor. In IOP situations with commercial insurance (where there is not a psychiatrist), the master's-level clinician would have to review with the MCO's physician.

The peer-to-peer review is usually a phone call between the patient's physician and the MCO's physician. The MCO's physician will generally lead the conversation and will render a decision at the end of the conversation as to whether or not more treatment will be covered.[16] Typically, when a case has gone peer to peer, it means that the MCO questions the validity of patient need or that the MCO does not want to pay for treatment.

The number of MCOs a clinician will deal with is based on the number of insurance network contracts the hospital or agency has. The MCOs vary in their policies and practices. Some MCOs are aggressive and demanding in their review habits in terms of both the frequency of review and the rigor of questioning. The stricter MCOs give shorter approval periods and are quicker to send cases for peer-to-peer review. Some MCOs routinely use peer-to-peer reviews, and their effects are reduced length of stays and increased denials.

THE CHALLENGES OF CONCURRENT
TREATMENT PLANNING

Besides dealing with the MCOs, there are a number of challenges to concurrent treatment planning. It is imperative that the clinician develop a working relationship with the hospital utilization review department. The clinician must have adequate organizational skills and flexibility when the utilization management department requests an abrupt review.[17] A successful clinician will have the interview and rapport skills to obtain the necessary information and to negotiate with the noncompliant

---

[16] In some peer-to-peer reviews, the MCO physician will tell the hospital physician or clinician at the beginning of the phone call that the request is denied without hearing any rationale for continued stay. Some MCOs have had a history of not approving PHP or IOP, with the blanket philosophy that the patient could be served in the regular outpatient setting and only become an inpatient if the patient becomes suicidal.

[17] Depending on how busy the in-house utilization reviewers and the clinician are, there may be an abrupt phone call that a patient is up for concurrent review and that additional information is required. The clinician should prepare a repertoire for such situations.

Fewer patients	More patients
More time available per patient	Less time available per patient
Fewer aggregate tasks	More aggregate tasks
More face-to-face interview time	Less availability for patient interviews
Less patient survey dependence	More patient survey dependence

Figure 4.1 *Workload tension based on patient census.*

patient. Part of the clinician's rapport skills is helping a patient identify when the patient is ready to return to work. Finally, the successful clinician will have good written and verbal communication skills. Appreciating these challenges is important for applying the appropriate strategies and accomplishing the treatment planning tasks.

On a given day, the clinician faces a continuum of task-oriented versus relational-oriented duties. Although necessary, the relational aspects take more time than the task-oriented duties. The emotionally needy patient may not appreciate the clinician's position that a higher patient census means more aggregate tasks that must be completed. The clinician will have a limited amount of time to complete tasks and need to seek as much efficiency as possible. Figure 4.1 shows this tension. The clinician will have to act in a task-oriented fashion while still maintaining tact and patient rapport to the extent that the patient is getting quality clinical service.[18]

Despite the need for efficiency, the clinician is dependent on a relationship with the utilization review department. He or she is expected to answer questions of the utilization review department as a job responsibility. The clinician often has to stop in the middle of other tasks and take phone calls or conduct impromptu patient interviews at the request of utilization reviewers.

The concurrent treatment planning interview can be challenging for the clinician if a patient evidences significant psychopathology and high acuity. If the patient has a high amount of anxiety, a significant portion of the interview may include calming the patient.[19] If the patient has a

---

[18] Clinicians in the PHP/IOP setting should consider their bedside manner as their expertise.

[19] An anxious patient's first question is often: "I'm not in any sort of trouble, am I?"

significant personality disorder such as narcissistic personality disorder or borderline personality disorder, he or she may find it difficult to focus. Such personality-disordered patients tend to be vague and nebulous in expressing problems, progress, and goals, and the interview can feel like a battle for control when the clinician is trying to gather all of the necessary information.[20] Even if the interview is not abrupt, a personality-disordered patient may avoid answering direct questions and digress to other subjects. The clinician is challenged to be soft but firm in keeping the patient focused on the task at hand.

Sometimes the patient demonstrates resistance or noncompliance to the treatment plan. When the clinician is reviewing the treatment plan progress, patients will report that they are not doing what was agreed upon. The clinician may also end up in a power struggle with the patient in this situation. In these cases, the clinician's challenge is to not work harder than the patient.

The last challenge to be discussed is that of communication by the clinician to the utilization reviewer and the MCO. The clinician should communicate effectively both verbally and in writing, expressing precisely the patient's need for continued treatment. The clinician should logically and succinctly report the patient's symptomology and effort expended in therapy.

The challenge is actually twofold as the clinician is also dependent on the utilization reviewer to communicate any peculiarities in MCO requests. Sometimes a rogue MCO care manager will insist on interventions or information that is not routine or within the scope of the program design.[21] Given the nature of the MCO reviewer's power, it is in the interest of the patient's treatment to attempt to satisfy the information request whenever possible. However, if the clinician is unaware of the particular

---

[20] If the clinician is getting an abrupt request from utilization management to get more information for concurrent review, then the clinician is incidentally making an abrupt request to talk to the patient. In such situations with personality-disordered patients, the clinician is often at the receiving end of the patient's resulting negative emotions and defensiveness.

[21] How a rogue MCO reviewer can make such demands is difficult to determine. There is typically no recourse when an MCO reviewer places stringent demands or refuses to give any consideration to clinical information.

requests of the MCO reviewer, the patient may have to be discharged before he or she is ready, regardless of the best efforts of the clinician and the patient's treatment compliance.[22]

THE GAME OF CONCURRENT TREATMENT PLANNING

Playing the game of concurrent treatment planning must take into account all the aforementioned challenges and actors. Furthermore, the clinician committed to mastering the job will work to reorganize priorities when the utilization review department calls, requesting immediate attention. In the beginning, the new clinician may feel like an improvisational comedy actor having to make up a routine on the spur of the moment in treatment planning. The strategies of concurrent treatment planning include:

- A basic evaluation and implementation process regarding data collection to minimize potential disruption to the work routine
- A daily commitment to the maintenance of a dashboard to track when a treatment plan review is to be conducted
- The development of several scripts for concurrent treatment planning

The next section discusses these strategies and their inherent tasks.

The Relationship With the Utilization Review Department

The strategies of evaluation and implementation processes include developing and maintaining a good relationship with the utilization department reviewers. An attitude of gaining mutual success should guide the interaction with the utilization review department.[23] Under the rubric of *internal customer,* the clinician and utilization manager can make each other's job easier. Some of this relationship development includes gaining an understanding of MCO styles and tendencies. The clinician

---

[22] Regardless of the MCO reviewer's demands, actual discharge is still dependent on the psychiatrist in the PHP and Medicare IOP situations.

[23] It is a healthy assumption that other employees want their jobs to go smoothly too.

and utilization reviewers can mutually develop an effective synergy that leads to longer patient stays, improved patient outcomes, and higher patient satisfaction.[24]

The clinician's contribution to this synergy includes implementation and routinization of information-gathering methods readily usable by the utilization reviewer. Such improvements can be made in interview scripts, patient surveys, and documentation styles. Effectively written clinical documentation and treatment plans can reduce additional requests for information, which further facilitates efficiency.

Organizational Routines

An essential part of clinician routine is a dashboard of review dates and end dates. A common software program such as Microsoft Outlook can prompt when treatment reviews are due. Another option is the creation and maintenance of a word-processing or spreadsheet file that tracks the pertinent patient information.[25] The form of such a document should include:

- Patient name
- Doctor (if applicable)
- Insurance/MCO name
- Admission date
- Treatment plan review date
- Patient-days approved
- Specific notes about the case (e.g., the insurance company/MCO is only giving so many days with the expectation to step down to outpatient status)

The clinician committing to this tool reviews and edits this document at the beginning and end of each day. Accordingly, he or she can make a work plan for the day and can forecast work plans for several days in advance.

---

[24] Furthermore, the clinician's good internal reputation with other organization employees goes a long way toward favorable cooperation from utilization reviewers in difficult cases.

[25] The dashboard document could be kept on paper, but it is recommended that it be maintained in a word-processing or spreadsheet program.

Interview Scripts

As noted earlier, the clinician has a combination of relational- and task-oriented duties. In light of the relational aspects of the job, the clinician may need to have two to three different work plans based on the foreseen workload. These scripts are based on (a) the functioning level of the patients to be interviewed, (b) how much the patient discloses in group therapy, and (c) the time available to complete the tasks.

Regardless of script form, the basic categories of patient information that the clinician is looking for are the same:

- What is the patient's progress?
- What is the patient's current symptomology?
- What is the patient's current functioning level?
- What are the patient's current goals or concerns?
- Does the patient feel ready for discharge?

If the patient is higher functioning, then the patient is more likely capable and willing to complete a survey or worksheet of assessment questions. On the other hand, if the patient either has lower intellectual functioning or is significantly symptomatic, or if the patient is an active participant in group therapy sessions, more information can be gleaned from the group therapy notes about the patient's current status and then through a face-to-face interview. Appendix B contains a list of review questions.

Script #1: The Patient Survey

The patient survey is the most efficient of the script options. The clinician can give a sheet of paper to the patient with all the pertinent questions and document the information in a patient note. However, the survey may run into problems when the patient does not or cannot answer all the questions. Furthermore, the survey is valid only to the extent that the patient is truthful and answers the questions fully. The survey is also subjective and does not give an objective opinion about a patient's affect. With the patient survey, faster is not always better.

Script #2: The Patient Interview

The patient interview refers to the clinician verbally asking all questions and recording the patient's answers. The patient interview is necessary when the patient obviously is more symptomatic or lower functioning. The clinician can observe the patient's mental status and affect. If the clinician has more time for the patient, then a full interview is acceptable, but this is not necessarily the best use of time as it can take more time than expected.

The following dialogue is based on the AIDET script. It is offered as an example of a concurrent treatment planning interview.

Dave: Hi Sally, I need to meet briefly with you to do treatment planning. I hope that within the next 10 minutes we can identify how you're currently doing, and where we need to go. Okay?

Sally: Okay.

Dave: How do you think you have improved since you started coming to our program?

Sally: I think I have done okay. I haven't been able to cook and we have been eating fast food. I still have problems getting to sleep and I can't stand to think about work. I haven't had thoughts of suicide for a few days. The group has helped me realize that I'm not alone.

Dave: Depression does have a way of making one feel all alone. Have you been taking the medication as prescribed?

Sally: Yes, I have been taking it. It is giving me a dull headache but the doctor told me that will go away.

Dave: Let's look at the goals that we agreed on last week. I have here that you were to take your medication, go for a walk daily, and talk in group about the relationship you were having with that difficult friend. I think I remember you talked about the difficult friend 2 days ago. You just said you were taking the medication, and you talked about the friend. Have you been taking the walks?

Sally: I have only walked 3 of the last 5 days.

Dave: Well, I think that you are still headed in the right direction. You have made some good efforts. What do we need to address more?

Sally: I still feel empty at times and I still feel like I am wearing a mask. There are times I feel that I just can't be who I am.

Dave: How about this? I suggest that you talk in the group about wearing a mask. I think that others in the group can relate to you. I also suggest that you talk about feeling emptiness. Others with depression feel that too, and I figure that you and the other group members can look for ways to find meaning and fulfillment. Will that work?

Sally: I think so.

Dave: Also, how about we keep the goals of taking medication and the effort to go for a daily walk?

Sally: I feel like I should be doing more.

Dave: This is depression. It is an illness. It makes things harder to do. But I offer a message of hope. It can get better. Okay, let's look at your current functioning. Using this depression scale where 0 means no depression and 10 means you are feeling suicidal, where is your depression?

Sally: Six.

Dave: Using the anxiety scale—where is yours today?

Sally: Five.

Dave: You said a minute ago that you did not have any thoughts of suicide for a little while. When was the last time you had those thoughts?

Sally: Yesterday.

Dave: Have you had any thoughts of wanting to hurt or kill someone?

Sally: Yes, but just my dead stepfather.

Dave: He is dead?

Sally: Yes, he died last year of cancer. I'm mad at him for how he beat my mother.

Dave: Thank you for telling me that. Have you been thinking about that all the time? Or does it come and go?

Sally: It comes and goes.

Dave: Sally, because of my time I am going to change gears on you even though you just mentioned something significant. You mentioned you haven't been getting sleep. How many hours a night are you getting?

Sally: About 5 hours.

Dave: What's normal?

Sally: About 7.

Dave: What's your appetite like?

Sally: Fair. I am eating about one meal and a snack each day. I eat here for lunch and maybe I have some fries when I get the fast food.

Dave: Sally, these questions are a little on the sensitive side, but I need to ask. Are you hearing any voices in your head that are not your voice?

Sally: No.

Dave: Are you seeing anything that others would say are not there?

Sally: I might be seeing some shadows.

Dave: Do you see them often?

Sally: No. It happens every few days.

Dave: Do you feel paranoid? Or that people are watching you or out to harm you?

Sally: I do feel that people are looking at me.

Dave: These are some other sensitive questions, but I need to ask. Have you used . . . or been using any alcohol or street drugs?

Sally: I've been pretty good about staying away from pot.

Dave: That means you haven't used it in the past week?

Sally: Yes, I have not used it in the past week.

Dave: Not trying to give you a morality lecture, but there is enough evidence indicating that it makes people depressed. I hope that you are able to stay away from it. Moving on . . . any new family stressors bothering you since you came to the program?

Sally: I have a sister telling me that I don't need medication and that I should just pull myself up by my bootstraps.

Dave: Do you think we need a family session with her to help out your recovery?

Sally: She lives in another state.

Dave: Any new legal or financial stressors?

Sally: I have had some bills that are coming that are worrying me, but if I can get back to work soon I will be okay.

Dave: Speaking of work, do you have any work-related concerns?

Sally: I want to go back to work when I am ready but I worry that people are going to come up to me and ask where I have been.

Dave: How much more time do you think you need here?

Sally: I suppose I need about another week.

Dave: Okay, let's move to when you are done here. I do not remember, but do you have a psychiatrist and therapist to go to?

Sally: No.

Dave: Do you want me to make an appointment for you?

Sally: Who would I go to?

Dave: Well, the default practice we refer to is the outpatient practice connected to the hospital. The usual plan is to start you off with a therapist and a physician. Most see the therapist for several sessions and see the physician on an ongoing basis.

Sally: How long will I see the doctor?

Dave: It varies for each patient, but the doctor usually wants to make sure your medication is at a therapeutic dose, wants to see an absence of symptoms for about 6 months, and then evaluates whether the dosage of your medication can be reduced and then slowly wean you off the medication.

Sally: How likely is that to happen?

Dave: Well, it is hard to say, but 9 out of 10 people with depression never have another episode. About 10% have to stay on medication longer. But there are many people out there who are taking psychiatric medication and we don't know it because it works in helping them live normal lives.

Sally: That is helpful. You can make the appointments for me.

Dave: That is all the information I need to cover. Are there any other issues or subjects that I have not brought up that you feel it is important for me to know about?

Sally: No.

Dave: Okay. I will report this to the insurance company, and I will see about getting you another week. See you tomorrow.

Script #3: The Combination Script and Interview

The combination of script and interview is probably the best for safety and risk management and can take less time than the interview alone. The patient can answer many of the interview questions regarding functioning on paper. The clinician can adjust the survey interview to focus interview questions where the pertinent issues lie. The clinician can get the subjective, self-report information faster and focus on objective observation in a briefer patient interview.

The degree to which a patient completes the survey is an indication of the patient's cognitive functioning and motivation. If the patient completes only about half the survey, the clinician can ask a question such as "I see the survey is only partially done. Did you have difficulty completing the survey?" The clinician can then make an appraisal about a patient's cognitive level, possible personality issues, or lack of motivation in treatment.

THE UNMOTIVATED PATIENT

There is a blurry line between acuity and malingering when it comes to the difficult patient who is not compliant in the PHP/IOP setting. Depending on the size of the clinician's caseload and therapy group, the noncompliant patient may not be as noticeable as in an outpatient setting.

One common situation of noncompliance in the PHP/IOP setting is the absent patient. From time to time, a patient will be absent from programming and will not answer the phone when staff call. The patient will then come back and not explain the absence. A patient may be absent to avoid issues. This may appear to be malingering, but in fact the patient may be too depressed to come to the program or answer the phone.

The frequency of absences has to be looked at within the context of the patient's work (or lack of work) in therapy.

Furthermore, in the PHP/IOP setting, the noncompliant patient at first may look acute because the clinician does not have a baseline. Patients may report that they have not worked on the goals because they feel they are just not well enough. However, after a few weeks of the same repeated pattern of absenteeism, it will appear that the patient is not compliant with treatment. The noncompliant patient may at first look acute, but time will tell whether it is a matter of acuity or malingering.[26]

In PHP/IOP settings where there is mandated family work, such as child/adolescent programs, the parental figures are often noncompliant with such sessions in a passive-aggressive manner. One example of this is that the child/adolescent will act as a messenger on the day of the scheduled session to report to the clinician that the parent cannot come to the family session (instead of the parent calling to reschedule). Also, the child/adolescent will be absent on the day of a scheduled family session. In both of these situations, the parent may not answer the phone when the clinician is calling to reschedule. In these cases, parents may want the child to change in the PHP/IOP, but are not willing to change themselves.[27]

When it comes to treatment noncompliance, the clinician has the danger of working harder than the patient. The clinician expects that the patient is going to attend, participate, and demonstrate improvement. The clinician also has some liability concerns and wants to minimize the risk of a suicidal patient. The clinician is working at an intense level with much acuity and wants to engage in appropriate clinical judgment and document that all clinical standards were met. Combining the acuity and intensity can lead the clinician to personalize inappropriately and worry or take inappropriate ownership of the patient's lack of progress.

---

[26] This situation is likely to occur in adult IOP settings with commercial insurance plans that do not have the required concurrent reviews. It can also occur in non-MCO settings such as U.S. Medicare or Medicaid.

[27] There are four typical scenarios in this case: (a) The stated problem is often that the child/adolescent has truancy issues and the family sees the program as an alternative to school; (b) the parent has psychopathology of his or her own, has no insight into his or her contribution to the family problem, and is reluctant to talk about change; (c) the parent is actively using substances; and (d) the parental figure is a foster parent and not interested in an emotional commitment to the child/adolescent. A family may demonstrate more than one of these scenarios.

The noncompliance gets complicated if a noncompliant patient in turn engages in staff splitting and instigation of drama after the clinician has interviewed the patient. Some noncompliant patients create neediness or crises that draw other staff members' attention to the patient. In this case, the needy patient makes critical statements of the assigned clinician that vaguely connote but do not substantiate incompetence. Such criticism tends to be emotional and subjective with no specific example of clinician behavior. PHP/IOP staff members who lack emotional intelligence and an appreciation of such patient behavior start to own the patient's emotions and problems and essentially work harder than the patient.

Not Working Harder Than the Patient

Not working harder than the noncompliant patient in the PHP/IOP setting is a commitment by the clinician to a principled approach that is cognizant of the structures within which the clinician must operate. The structures include the following:

- The clinician has to abide by the policy regarding when a patient is discharged.
- Most payer sources expect compliance and monitor symptomology.
- Most payer sources will not certify more days if someone is not compliant with the treatment.
- If the patient does not attend, the system does not consider that the patient needs the services.
- Treatment eventually has to end and the patient cannot stay forever.

Sometimes the clinician must patiently detach and tolerate a noncompliant patient while documenting that all reasonable clinical efforts were made.

Part of the patience required with the noncompliant patient is the use of soft skills in which the clinician affirms limits and choices. Often, the noncompliant patient presents himself or herself as a victim without choices. The clinician may need to act confused along with the helpless patient about not knowing what to. The clinician then affirms that the PHP/IOP has limits as to what the program can do for a patient. The clinician may need to state some of the structures listed previously by which the clinician is bound. This approach is soft, yet firm.

CONCLUSIONS

This chapter discussed the game of concurrent treatment planning. It is an unexciting but necessary game for the PHP/IOP clinician to master. It is a challenging game given the intensity of a PHP/IOP milieu and the demands of managed care. However, playing this game well will likely mean positive economic externalities that include longer patient stays, a higher daily census, more effective treatment, and higher patient satisfaction.

The PHP/IOP clinician who is successful at the game of concurrent treatment planning will demonstrate a mix of task-oriented and relational-oriented strategies to achieve getting the necessarily clinical data. The clinician will need to build bridges of cooperation with the in-house utilization reviewers. The clinician will also need to develop and polish organization and time management skills in concurrent treatment planning to work smarter and not harder to combine efficiency and clinical effectiveness.

The clinical data elements that concurrent treatment planning seeks to gather are routine in the typical case. The conditions under which the information elements must be gathered vary based on patient census and patient acuity. A higher census will mean a tendency toward task-oriented approaches, whereas a higher level of acuity will require more relational-oriented approaches. The suggested task-oriented approach is a paper survey and the suggested relational approach is the patient interview. The clinician will need a strategy of at least three approaches of concurrent treatment planning, utilizing a paper survey and a verbal interview to balance task and relational needs.

The clinician cannot work harder than the unmotivated patient. There is a general assumption that PHP/IOP is an intense treatment setting that is not a normal life situation for the patient. It is expected that PHP/IOP patients appreciate that they are in a crisis or near-crisis situation that requires intense focus on treatment so as to return to a regular life.[28] Although a clinician often needs to guide a patient toward realistic treatment goals, the patient either works on the treatment goals or does

---

[28] This expectation is generally relaxed for the serious mentally ill and geriatric patients as they do not necessarily have an expectation of returning to work or school.

not. The clinician is part of a systemic structure that has limits and expectations, and if a patient proves to be noncompliant, the payment system will move for discharge from treatment. The clinician is more effective acting as a polite but firm messenger of this reality versus trying to parent a noncompliant or unmotivated patient; it is nothing personal—it is just the way the system works.

Sometimes the unmotivated or noncompliant patient may try to punish the limit-setting clinician by complaining to the other staff that the clinician is "pushy" or "expecting too much" of the patient. Although a clinician may engage in introspection in these situations, it helps to look at the bigger picture: The majority of PHP/IOP patients comply with treatment and want to get well.

As a PHP/IOP clinician continues to play the game of concurrent treatment planning and gains experience, it can become evident how the clinician can be more efficient while maintaining effectiveness. Good concurrent treatment planning requires evaluation, identification of where improvement can be made, and the implementation of those changes.

REFERENCES

Berger, S. (2002). *Fundamentals of health care financial management: A practical guide to financial issues and activities* (2nd ed.). San Francisco, CA: Jossey-Bass.
MacKenzie, R. (Ed.). (1995). *Effective use of group therapy in managed care.* Washington, DC: American Psychiatric Press.

CHAPTER FIVE

DISCHARGE PLANNING

Termination refers to the end of the psychotherapist–patient relationship in the outpatient treatment setting. The door is theoretically open, should the patient wish to return to address more issues. The terminating patient has likely achieved the maximum progress, and treatment can stop.[1]

In the higher levels of the treatment continuum, *discharge* refers to when it is time to end treatment. It is expected that the patient has not resolved all of his or her pertinent issues and will need some form of follow-up treatment at a lower level of care. Patient follow-up may include arranging for other services or giving the patient instructions to make certain appointments. *Discharge planning* includes the set of activities of arranging a patient's follow-up treatment and is the term used in the partial hospitalization program (PHP)/intensive outpatient program (IOP) setting.

At face value, discharge planning in the PHP/IOP seems to be a simple act of contacting outpatient providers for a patient or agreeing with a patient that he or she will make the appropriate appointments. However, discharge planning from the PHP/IOP setting can be challenging.

A number of writers have used the term *regional preferences* to refer to the local differences in PHP/IOP services. It is held here that regional preferences are really the political–economic realities of each locality.[2] These political–economic realities create challenges for discharge planning.[3]

---

[1] The patient can also decide he or she just does not want any more treatment, regardless of the continued symptoms or recommendation of the clinician for treatment to continue.

[2] In this context, *preferences* connotes that there is a rational decision-making process. Instead, there are both political and economic tensions between interests that produce the local or regional options.

[3] As part of the political–economic realities, a PHP/IOP service can exist only if there is both the political will and the market capacity for it. An organization must see an economic opportunity, have the support of key stakeholders, and be willing to take the financial risk to implement the PHP/IOP services.

This chapter discusses discharge planning as a game in a generalized sense that is applicable to different cohorts.[4] It is written with the assumption that the clinician is required to make the aftercare appointment for the patient.[5] This chapter discusses the political–economic challenges of discharge planning and then suggests a game of practical strategies.

POLITICAL ECONOMY CHALLENGES

Within the structure of federal and state laws and policies,[6] numerous political–economic influences are a hegemonic reality in each locality. These influences are commercial insurance, public insurance, employee assistance program (EAP) providers, psychiatrists, treatment cohorts, and the provider organization. These influences also include government interests; corporate interests outside of the local area; and vested, local interests that control available options for discharge planning. A clinician who has an appreciation of the local political–economic interests can negotiate the aftercare system more effectively in discharge planning. This section reviews the general categories of these challenging influences.

---

[4] This will be discussed again in Chapters 9, 10, 11, 12, and 13.

[5] As is discussed later, due to managed care organization (MCO) pressure, the patient's appointments typically must be made at the time of discharge, which places the onus on the clinician. Some practices and agencies require the patient or family to make the appointments with the practice directly. The rationale varies, but the most common reason is that a patient will be more likely to keep the appointment if the patient or parent makes it instead of a clinician or discharge planner.

[6] Localities are not sovereign like nation–states (Peterson, 1981). In terms of "urban political economy," they are not the sum of the state or local government either. Localities exist within the rules and structure allowed by higher levels of government. In the case of the United States, state and federal laws lay down provisions and processes. In terms of local health care structure, additional structure exists due to accreditation organizations. The accreditation organizations have quasigovernmental power to impose structure as allowed by federal rules.

Insurance

The payer sources in a locality influence many discharge options. Berger (2002) noted that the health insurance system has separated the consumer from the health care buying decision. A patient rarely makes a rational choice in the amount or level of product consumption (p. xiii). The typical insured patient who cannot pay the cash rate for services is limited to the relevant providers available in a locality.

Commercial Insurance

Within the commercial insurance sector, there is an appearance of economic control on both the supply side and the demand side. The hegemony theoretically keeps health care costs down.

This economic hegemony occurs in many U.S. localities because major employers buy insurance packages or plans for their employees from a limited number of carriers.[7] There is an economic logic that there will be employee demand for health care providers who take the particular insurance plan.

The insurance carriers in turn control the economic supply through the creation of "panels" or networks of health care providers to include psychiatrists and therapists of various credentials. A condition of being in the network includes a contractual obligation to accept a specific reimbursement rate and charge the patient a specific copay amount.[8,9] The managed care organizations discourage patients from choosing providers outside of the network.[10]

As part of the hegemony, MCOs or insurance carriers may cue the PHP/IOP clinician on discharge plans. The cue may include a time frame

---

[7] Government (local, state, federal) units in the United States are also major employers that use larger commercial insurance carriers along with the carrier's network or panel.

[8] The provider contract also includes precertification and utilization review policies.

[9] Berger (2002, p. 11) notes that the copayment is a managed care tool to discourage the utilization of services.

[10] The higher copay or out-of-pocket expense discourages a patient from using a provider out of the network.

by which aftercare appointments are made with network providers. An MCO may issue some statement-of-quality review, grading how well a hospital has performed in terms of following the discharge-planning cues.[11]

Public Insurance (Medicaid/Medicare[12])

With regard to public insurance in the United States, the discharge-planning options are typically more limited than are those used with commercial insurance. The lower reimbursement rates and arduous enrollment requirements discourage many from becoming Medicare and Medicaid providers.[13] The community mental health agency may be the Medicaid and Medicare recipient's only local choice. [14,15]

Therefore, when the patient has Medicaid or Medicare, the discharge planning from PHP/IOP is practically predetermined. If the attending psychiatrist does not take Medicaid or Medicare in an outpatient practice,

---

[11] The quality scores or ratings could have implications for the renewal of the organization's contract with the insurance carrier.

[12] It is noted that Canada and the United States both have programs called *Medicare*. In the United States, *Medicare* is for either the elderly or the disabled. In Canada, *Medicare* is the encompassing title for the national health insurance program; http://www.hc-sc.gc.ca/hcs-sss/medi-assur/index-eng.php. Further references to *Medicare* refer to the U.S. setting.

[13] Furthermore, a therapist in private practice taking Medicaid or Medicare must practice under the supervision of a psychiatrist, which also limits opportunities.

[14] The local mental health agency is largely constrained by numerous federal laws ultimately tied to funding.

[15] Some larger urban areas may have additional Medicaid and Medicare outpatient providers such as a medical school with an outpatient clinic for teaching purposes, but patient choices are still more limited than with commercial insurance. Some patients who have been previously served at community mental health agencies are dissatisfied with those services and resist referrals back to those entities. The clinician often has to attend to the patient's resistance and explore what options exist. If a patient does not want to return to the community mental health agency, the clinician should document that this was processed with the patient.

the patient will have to follow up with outpatient providers who do take Medicaid or Medicare.

Whether involving public or private insurance, the PHP/IOP implication of the limitations is that the average patient will have relatively few choices for outpatient mental health services. A patient with commercial insurance who has the finances to pay cash to any provider he or she wants is generally the exception. The PHP/IOP clinician will often have to educate the patient with insurance on how the transition to outpatient services works.

Employee Assistance Programs

Because they are referral sources, EAPs can be powerful influences in discharge planning. Larger employers, including governments, often contract with EAPs that are either individual clinicians or corporations to provide a continuum of services that encompass counseling and sensitivity training. Some EAP providers serve as the MCO for an insurance plan and engage in utilization management. EAP responsibilities include determining whether an employee is fit to return to work.

Some EAP providers will be intimately involved in discharge planning, whereas others just want a phone call when a patient is to be discharged. Clinician mindfulness of the different modus operandi of the EAP providers is important in quality patient care and effective time management.

Interacting with the EAP often requires diplomatic tact. An EAP is in the power position when it is both the referral source and decision maker about a patient's return to work. When a patient avoids contact with the EAP, the clinician can be thrown into a triangle of drama with these two; and therefore the clinician will need to practice clear, consistent boundaries with the EAP and the patient.

The Treatment Cohort

The patient cohort also has implications for outpatient services. Psychiatry and other outpatient therapies are diverse with subspecialties. Although the community mental health agency will usually serve both adults and children with Medicare and Medicaid, regardless of specialized needs, many other outpatient providers taking commercial insurance serve either just adults or just children.

Discharge planning for specialty cohort areas such as gerontology, addiction, or eating disorders can be challenging. Although larger metropolitan areas typically have more specialty providers because the market supports them, a clinician in smaller cities may have to merely identify the provider best qualified who may not be a specialist in the needed area. Another challenge exists when an MCO insists that a patient be referred to a provider who is not reputable in a specialty.[16] An ethical matter evolves into a political–economic issue when there are no available specialists in a specific locality or an MCO insists on its discharge plan.

The Psychiatrist

The psychiatrist is at the top of the proverbial food chain and has the final decision in the discharge-planning process. In a typical PHP situation, which requires a psychiatrist, the psychiatrist orders the admission and discharge.[17,18] The psychiatrist chooses whether to refer a patient to the psychiatrist's outpatient practice or to another provider. The clinician is obligated to follow the psychiatrist's discharge order under the risk of sanction, discipline, or termination.

Psychiatrists have different attitudes when it comes to insurance/ MCO mandates to discharge a patient. Some unequivocally discharge a patient when an MCO cues it, whereas others regularly go "peer to peer." Appreciating these different preferences of psychiatrists is helpful both in time management and in advising a patient on the discharge process.

Psychiatrists also vary in the object of their discharge instructions. Some expect clinicians to make the aftercare appointments, whereas others measure motivation by requiring patients or guardians to call the office.

---

[16] If an outpatient provider engages in misrepresentation as a specialist in a field, then a clinician may wish to consult the appropriate state licensing board and available codes of ethical conduct and decide whether a complaint is in order.

[17] Some hospitals have administrative discharge procedures in cases of disruptive patient behavior, regardless of the psychiatrist's choice not to discharge a patient.

[18] Commercial insurance does not require a psychiatrist for a patient in the IOP setting. Medicare does require a psychiatrist at the IOP level. A psychiatrist may be consulted for a medication check for an IOP patient and in turn may order a particular discharge plan.

When the patient or guardian is supposed to make the appointments, the clinician may get phone calls from MCOs and utilization review personnel asking for aftercare information he or she does not have.[19]

Psychiatric practices vary in the sophistication of the organization and procedural details followed for making appointments. Larger practices tend to have specialized intake staff, whereas smaller practices have generalists handling multiple duties. It is useful for a clinician to research the psychiatry practices he or she frequently calls to understand these differences in order to make aftercare duties flow in a smooth and efficient manner.[20]

The Organization

Other than the psychiatrist's prerogative, the hospital or agency may also have discharge-planning rules. The organization rules typically apply when the psychiatrist is a hospitalist, or the patient was only in the IOP with commercial insurance.[21] Such policy may be codified, exist as management instruction, or merely be organizational habit. More often than not, the organization rules apply to clinician self-referral and to when the organization has an outpatient practice of its own.

The Clinician With a Private Practice

A PHP/IOP clinician with a private practice on the side can be a political–economic influence in discharge planning, but there are some risks. The clinician in this situation faces greater scrutiny over the appearance of

---

[19] In the name of serving internal customers, it is favorable to attempt to fulfill utilization review requests and then document the attempts.

[20] When building linkages with the practices, it is a helpful strategy to ask how the clinician can make the intake process easier for the practice staff. If the clinician can routinize those requested steps, it will likely speed up the scheduling of aftercare and increase the likelihood that the appointments are received the same day.

[21] The hospitalist psychiatrist may or may not be a hospital employee. The hospitalist may be obligated to refer to the organization outpatient practice when in existence.

a conflict of interest.[22] The clinician may lose a patient when a psychiatrist orders a discharge to the psychiatrist's practice and associated therapists.[23]

Patient Choice as It Exists

In the end, the patient or guardian always has self-determination whether to comply with treatment. The patient and/or guardian can choose not to follow the discharge-planning recommendations with all of the implications and consequences of refusing the recommendations, whether they are psychiatric, job related, relational, or legal.[24,25]

Summary

Successful discharge planning for a patient takes into account the political–economic realities of care. The political–economic realities of a locality limit existing follow-up choices. Quality patient care includes advising the patient or guardian on these limits in cases of dissatisfaction with discharge recommendations. Although the PHP/IOP clinician cannot be responsible for the guardian or patient's choice, the clinician is responsible for clearly documenting that the discharge-planning efforts were made.

---

[22] The clinician will have to ensure that the prior relationship is documented somewhere in the medical record. It would be best if the admitting department could document this at the time of intake.

[23] In these cases, the psychiatrist has a practice with associated therapists and a rule that the patient must see those therapists. Some psychiatrists do not fully review the chart or assessment documents and are ignorant of a preexisting relationship. It is in the clinician's interest to declare the preexisting relationship to the psychiatrist.

[24] Consequences can include loss of job, significant relationship, or loss of custody of children.

[25] The legal system is often a referral source for a patient. Typically, the patient must produce some kind of statement that he or she is compliant or has completed treatment. Some patients get incarcerated because they do not comply with treatment.

THE GAME OF DISCHARGE PLANNING

The game of discharge planning involves relationships and a set of efficient measures. The successful clinician will make discharge appointments while getting other work done. The successful clinician will have organizational and efficiency strategies in place to facilitate successful aftercare appointment scheduling and to meet documentation needs.

Given that all PHP/IOP programs have a limited number of practicing psychiatrists and aftercare options, the clinician should research the policies and procedures of the outpatient practices and develop an effective and efficient routine of discharge procedures. The development of the routine also includes building a synergistic relationship with the practice so a win–win is achieved.[26] The resultant routine will include knowing the best times to call the outpatient practices and sending faxes, when possible, versus waiting for return phone calls.[27]

The practice of faxing requests for appointments is more effective when practices are busy or have fewer people to answer the phone. When faxing information to psychiatric offices, typed documents are preferable because handwriting can be unclear. When possible, the development of word-processing templates for faxes is an effective organizational strategy to use.[28]

Prioritization plays into organizational strategy. Although it is up to the clinician to determine what works for him or her, making aftercare appointments should be considered a priority over most other clinical tasks. The following is a suggested prioritization of tasks:

- A clinician should first ensure the safety of a suicidal or homicidal patient.
- A clinician's second responsibility is to conduct a scheduled group therapy session.

---

[26] Knowing the names of the office staff and calling them by name is an effective relational tool.

[27] The clinician should research organizational policies on the use of faxes and e-mails, as organizations have different standards on the communication of protected health information.

[28] This strategy is possible when the clinician has an available computer and data storage.

- Making discharge appointments for a patient should be a third priority.
- Concurrent treatment planning with a patient should be a fourth priority.

The logic of this prioritization is that safety is first and milieu management is second. However, a caveat is that the intensity of the work and the needs of other patients can easily distract the clinician from making aftercare appointments. Scheduling aftercare appointments as far in advance as possible makes for less frustration and greater satisfaction for all the relevant interests.[29]

If the appointments cannot be made by the time the programming is over for the day, the appointment should be made by the end of the business day. Appointments should be made by the end of the next business day at the latest. The likelihood of appointments getting made diminishes with time.

Developing a routine for making appointments does involve some research and experimentation with methods. The research involves talking with the psychiatrists and their office staff about policies and preferences. The experimentation has to do with creating methods and documents for effectively contacting the psychiatry practices and agencies to schedule the patient appointments.

LETTERS FOR WORK AND SCHOOL

In addition to making the appointments, a clinician receives requests from patients and families for letters or "doctor's notes" to substantiate treatment. Typically, the note must be signed by a physician, but the request is made to the clinician. The note can be on a prescription pad, or it can be in the form of a letter. The form depends on the psychiatrist's preference and the specificity of the employer's or EAP's requirements.

The letter or note should be brief but pleasant in tone. The letter should be dated and indicate that the patient was discharged on a specific date. It should have a statement that the patient is released to return

---

[29] Some practices will make appointments only on the day of discharge.

to work or school or is expected to be out for a certain period of time.[30] The clinician can choose to include a line indicating contact information if there are further questions. A copy of the letter should be placed in the medical record.

The clinician can easily organize the task of letter writing by creating word-processing templates that are electronically saved. There should be at least one template for each practicing psychiatrist in the program.[31] If a particular EAP or large employer is represented frequently in the patient census, then the clinician should also create a template reflecting those interests. A good template should use software settings to automatically set the date. The letter should be printed on the organization's letterhead.[32] Appendix C offers an example of a template for discharge purposes.

CONCLUSIONS

This chapter discussed discharge planning for the PHP/IOP setting in a manner intended to be generalized and applicable to all cohorts. At face value, discharge planning in the PHP/IOP setting appears to be a simple task, but it can be a source of frustration and disruption when the clinician is trying to juggle multiple tasks and problems. Discharge planning can be complex, based on the requirements and parameters of organizational policy, the different payer sources, referral sources, and aftercare resources.

There are common political–economic challenges that a clinician must take into account when doing discharge planning. Although the

---

[30] In this writer's experience, some employers have asked for a letter that says a patient is not going to have any future episodes and is safe to return to work. Any such letters can reflect only a patient's stability on a given date. A psychiatrist cannot predict future episodes.

[31] Numerous templates can be created based on gender pronouns and various degrees of information. However, when a clinician spends more than a few minutes searching for the most appropriate choice, there are probably too many templates.

[32] An organization's (especially a psychiatric hospital's) letterhead connotes influence, which should result in being readily accepted by the receiving party.

patient is a consumer or customer, the political–economic reality in discharge planning can make the patient appear to be merely an economic commodity, yielding revenue from copayments and insurance payments. In each locality or region, the mental health "system" has a number of interests or players with vested economic and political stakes in mental health services. The interplay of the interests creates the sum of local preferences through bargaining and influence. Where a clinician refers a patient for aftercare treatment is predetermined by these political–economic realities.

Helpful time management and organizational techniques for clinicians in this area take some research and preparation. Ascertaining practice referral preferences makes for a smoother process. The clinician can use that preference information to create routine templates for making appointments and brief doctor notes. Such efficiency in discharge planning allows a clinician to successfully prioritize and balance work tasks in the intense PHP/IOP practice situation.

REFERENCES

Berger, S. (2002). *Fundamentals of health care financial management: A practical guide to financial issues and activities* (2nd ed.). San Francisco, CA: Jossey-Bass.

Peterson, P. E. (1981). *City limits*. Chicago, IL: University of Chicago Press.

CHAPTER SIX

GROUP THERAPY

Group therapy is the primary treatment modality across all the partial hospitalization program (PHP)/intensive outpatient program (IOP) settings; group therapy allows the therapist to work efficiently with several patients at one time. Group therapy skills are essential for a clinician working in the PHP/IOP setting.

This chapter is written with three assumptions. It first assumes that the reader has graduated from a clinical program with a curriculum in group therapy, as this chapter does not provide a comprehensive review on the subject.[1] A second assumption is that a PHP/IOP has its group sessions within a 3- to 4-hour time frame. Third, the group combines PHP and IOP clients and contains patients with different levels of acuity. The assumptions tend to limit this chapter's value to process group therapy in adult cohorts.[2]

Similar to the inpatient setting, the process group in the PHP/IOP setting is an open group with a high degree of turnover with frequent admissions and discharges.[3] It differs from the inpatient setting in that the group is the main therapeutic element and not one of several treatment modalities. It is not like the typical outpatient group where the patients are referred for a specific problem and screened for the ability to participate; the PHP/IOP patients are diverse, and admission is based on

---

[1] The book by Yalom and Leszcz (2005) is good for a review of group therapy theory. Any of Yalom's previous editions of this book are also excellent.

[2] Some PHPs (especially child and adolescent) operate similarly to inpatient units where the program runs all day and groups are interspersed with other activities.

[3] The stream of movement in and out of a group varies and the rate of group turnover is generally unpredictable.

meeting the acuity criteria for the specific level of care.[4] The clinician is challenged daily to lead a diverse collection of strangers into a therapeutic group that benefits each of the patients.

Group therapy in the PHP/IOP setting has a different therapeutic value and function across the different cohorts. However, one consistent function is that the patients will be monitored for safety and symptomology due to higher acuity. Adult patients can benefit through self-disclosure and giving feedback. Child groups emphasize socialization, expression of feelings, and the development of basic coping skills. Adolescent and preadolescent groups will vary in approach and accomplishment based on the acuity, cognitive development, and maturity levels of the patients.[5] Not all cohorts are capable of benefiting from group therapy in the same manner.

Regardless of the cohort, group therapy has great therapeutic potential in the PHP/IOP setting. When intensely acute patients realize they are not alone in their problems, they tend to develop hope, acceptance, and validation, which in turn can reduce anxiety and depressive symptoms. The patients appear to have greater credibility at times than clinicians because of having experienced existentially the same symptoms and issues. Besides symptom alleviation, groups give patients opportunities to gain insight and demonstrate personal competence.[6]

The PHP/IOP clinician is not a passive observer who waits to see whether a therapeutic group spontaneously forms. The clinician is a catalyst who initiates interactions about therapeutic matters that should facilitate self-disclosure and give feedback. In the face of the symptoms of depression and anxiety, the clinician is a normative emotional barometer

---

[4] One exception is screening geriatric adults for dementia. Federal regulations require that if a patient has dementia, it must be mild and the patient must retain the ability to remember from one session to another.

[5] Functioning considerations in the case of adolescents includes maturity level, cognitive functioning, and symptomology. Some adolescent groups will consist of more mature and cognitive individuals whereas some groups will consist of immature and disruptive patients.

[6] For adults, the competence is in being able to help other adults with suggestions and knowledge. In child groups, the child gets rewarded for good behavior and is praised for appropriate behavior. Competence in adolescent groups varies between the intrinsic rewards gained by adults and praise from the clinician.

who guides patients to rational thinking, normal emotional reaction, and healthy behavioral patterns. How the clinician leads, guides, and manages the group makes a difference in patient safety, patient retention, and patient satisfaction.[7]

This chapter discusses the game of process group therapy at the PHP/IOP level of care in general terms. It explores the general limits and challenges of process group therapy at this level of care.[8] It then discusses a game of basic strategies for dealing with the challenges in starting and maintaining a process group. Finally, suggestions for dealing with common group problems are presented.

CHALLENGES AND LIMITS TO GROUP THERAPY IN THE PHP/IOP SETTING

As an open group, the IOP/PHP group has limits in what can be discussed and addressed. It is a heterogeneous group containing relatively acute and fragile patients coming from different backgrounds and possessing different needs. For various reasons, the patients will not all participate to an equal degree in the group. Furthermore, the clinician has the challenge of multitasking in the course of a group session. This section discusses these challenges and limits.

The Open Group

The PHP/IOP group will have a limited ethos. The patient turnover diminishes the likelihood of intimacy found in the typical closed outpatient group. On the whole, the patients are admitted to address acuity rather than a specific issue, and the acuity itself may be the only commonality on some days. Acuity, especially anxiety, in itself is a barrier to being in a group of strangers. In addition to acuity, stigmas about

---

[7] Two helpful analogies are (a) the clinician is a dance instructor actively teaching the dance of group process, and (b) the clinician is actively teaching the patients how to play a game.

[8] Other types of groups used with children and adolescents are discussed in Chapter 12.

needing psychiatric treatment in the first place engender paralysis in patients toward group participation. The clinician therefore frequently has the challenge of creating an ethos of acceptance and connection in the midst of intense acuity, stigma, and diversity.

Acuity and Diversity

Besides the issues of ethos, the social diversity within the patient cohorts and the acuity of the patients can challenge group order and focus. Given the crisis nature of PHP/IOP admission, patient diversity is theoretically irrelevant. It can stay irrelevant and likely unknown as long as the group members have found enough commonality and tolerance to focus on treatment. Diversity's challenges to a group's therapeutic focus are not discovered until they become the root of a group conflict or problem. The clinician is thus challenged to negotiate and mediate conflicts arising from diversity and to keep the group therapeutically focused.

As discussed in Chapter 1, acuity reduces a patient's functioning, which suggests that admission to a therapy group of strangers is an additional stress. The acute patient tends to have increased anxiety and less ability to participate in new situations. Such patients tend to have more anxiety when talking about themselves and in response to the reactions they receive from other group participants.[9]

In light of patient acuity, the diversity of the PHP/IOP group also limits the subjects that can be safely discussed. An acute patient may have less cognitive ability and distress tolerance, which makes participation in abstract and controversial topics difficult. Intimate subjects such as trauma, sexual issues, and religion are inherently stressful to discuss and tend to require trust and connection not necessarily present in the group at any given time. Discussion of sex and trauma can trigger flashbacks that evolve into suicidal ideation in acute patients.[10] Some patients may simply be so offended by the insensitivity in the discussion that they

---

[9] The anxious patients may have cognitive distortions that may need to be challenged in the course of the treatment.

[10] Flashbacks are stressful memories that can overwhelm an acute patient. The patient can become suicidal because he or she cannot cope with the feelings, and that patient may need admission or readmission as an inpatient.

do not return for treatment without notice.[11] In order to maintain a safe therapeutic environment, the clinician is challenged to maintain mindfulness about the group composition and redirect patients to bringing up intimate topics when appropriate.[12]

The challenge of maintaining a safe group environment includes managing patient anger outbursts. Although depression and anxiety can underlie irritability and anger, outbursts tend to produce a chilling effect that detracts from the treatment of other patients. Some patients may engage in personal attacks on other patients.[13] Context does matter, as some patients may be appropriately intense when engaged in self-disclosure. However, an irritable patient habitually using profanity may degrade safety, as other anxious group members cannot tolerate the anger. The clinician and treatment team are challenged to demonstrate composure, control, and perspective in order to minimize patient disruption through the continued pursuit of a therapeutic group process.[14]

Unequal Participation

Even if a group is safe, not all PHP/IOP patients participate equally due to personal issues, acuity, and personality type. Many patients have never been in group therapy before and have no experience about talking about their feelings and issues in a group setting. Some patients have

---

[11] Heterosexual discussion of sexual issues can be offensive to gay and lesbian group members.

[12] Adult therapy groups may evolve into homogeneous gender groups where the patients have been in attendance for several days. Also, when a mixed-gender group has been left intact for several days, it may have developed significant bonds. The group in either situation may manifest the safety, trust, and motivation to discuss difficult subjects.

[13] This is discussed further in Chapter 14.

[14] A new clinician taking over an established group may see a cabal form. The cabal forms when the group consists of significant psychopathology and has been emotionally attached to the exiting therapist. The cabal members are mad and feel abandoned because the exiting clinician is leaving. The new therapist is the object of anger. In these cases, it is important for a clinician to collaborate with the treatment team and supervisor to manage the situation with an eye toward reestablishing a therapeutic milieu.

stressors that are only appropriate for individual therapy.[15] Introverted patients are less inclined to talk in group settings. On the other hand, a patient evidencing codependent traits or low self-esteem may refuse to speak out of the belief that the other patients have more serious problems and deserve all the group time. Patients with agoraphobia or social anxiety may also be withdrawn in group sessions due to intense anxiety.[16] Although there is no guarantee that these patients will talk more, the clinician is challenged to make a mindful effort to create an open and accepting environment that prompts patients to talk.

Group therapy also varies in its effectiveness due to patient behavior and symptomology, which vary from day to day. In the process of recovery (see Figure 1.2 in Chapter 1), patients may have temporarily regressed, but regain improvement 1 to 2 days later. When patients have managed symptoms and are orderly in their behavior, group therapy participation by all group members is more likely. However, a manic patient presenting with grandiosity and euphoria may be insensitive to the social cues from anxious patients in the group.[17] A psychotic patient may be responding to internal stimuli such as visual or auditory hallucinations and be disconnected from the group and reality in general. Group symptomology affects what can be discussed in group therapy and the number of patients who will participate.

Motivational Differences

The patient's motivation also has implications for group participation. Despite the stigma of seeking treatment, the average patient is sufficiently

---

[15] A clinician may ascertain that a PHP/IOP group may have a high concentration of acute, insensitive, or immature group members who are incapable of handling an intimate issue. Also, if a person's main stressor is being accused of sexual abuse, he or she should not be discouraged from discussing that issue in the group due to the likelihood of abuse survivors being present in the group. In this case, there is a risk of significantly disrupting the group with multiple discharges because the survivors do not feel safe.

[16] Agoraphobic patients may have poor program attendance in the first place.

[17] The manic patient may be grandiose or talk about inappropriate subjects. Furthermore, the mania may be a surprise as a patient may come in reporting that he or she is there for depression, and in the course of treatment, it is evident that the patient manifests the criteria for a diagnosis of bipolar disorder.

motivated to be in the program to resolve symptoms or to avoid some consequence.[18] Although severely depressed patients may not present as being motivated and active in the group, they tend to comply quietly with the order of the milieu. An unmotivated patient presenting as both anxious and irritable can undermine group dynamics through consistent but challenging and sarcastic help rejection. A "junior therapist" will make frequent prescriptions for other group members while avoiding his or her own problems. An adolescent with attention deficit hyperactivity disorder who refuses to take his or her medication may talk on the side, distract others, or act out impulsively during group therapy because of the inability to focus. Acuity challenges the clinician to minimize the distraction of unmotivated patients in the group.

Monitoring the Group as Individual Patients

In addition to managing patient challenges, the PHP/IOP clinician must simultaneously juggle monitoring patient acuity while directing the group to focus on germane therapeutic topics.[19] Such documentation of patient acuity and participation is expected to be thorough and directly relevant to the patient's treatment plan. Depending on the program organization, the clinician's group note may bear crucial weight as the sole clinical documentation on a given day.[20]

The Limits of Group Therapy

In addition to the aforementioned challenges, group therapy in the PHP/IOP setting has inherent limits related to patient choice. To benefit,

---

[18] There are a number of potential consequences in these cases. For adults, these include probation violations, conditions of employment, and conditions required to maintain professional licensure. For children and adolescents, the potential consequences are incarceration and foster care placement.

[19] In the inpatient setting, there are multiple staff members with various credentials who document patient behaviors over the course of a day.

[20] The weight of the note is also related to the level of acuity a patient has. Otherwise, in the inpatient setting, the weight of the documentation is spread among the disciplines.

a patient needs to participate in the group through self-disclosure and feedback. Because they are not professionals, there is a risk that group members may give inaccurate, inappropriate, or unsupportive feedback to others. Third, as discussed in previous chapters, a patient is admitted for a relatively short time based on acuity, and so chronic problems will likely be unresolved in the program. Furthermore, although the group can support a patient with helpful insight and suggested alternatives, the patient must take responsibility for his or her own recovery.

Another inherent limit of group therapy is that it will not attend to all the needs of all the patients. Fortunately, many of the patients will evidence sufficient maturity to appreciate their responsibility for meeting personal needs. The clinician may have to review these limits with the patients in group and treatment planning conferences.

Summary of Limits and Challenges

Understanding the challenges and limits is necessary for organizing and running a productive process therapy group at the PHP/IOP level. With all of the inherent challenges, a clinician is essentially confronting a different puzzle every day as to the patient composition of the group. In solving the puzzle, the clinician is objectively attempting to create an environment, which increases the likelihood that patients will gain a therapeutic benefit and be accurately monitored for safety and acuity.

THE GAME OF THE GROUP PROCESS

Given all the challenges and limits, the game of group therapy in the PHP/IOP setting is essentially task oriented in nature and guides the patients in treatment. The clinician is an active and directive group leader who will provide structure to the group sessions to gather the clinical information required by the managed care organizations (MCOs) and catalyze therapeutic group dynamics. The clinician also will seek to be an influential director outside of the group in individual treatment planning sessions with patients in providing guidance about group participation. As a subset of the program's therapeutic milieu, the therapy group should be a structured experience that provides as much stability as possible in the midst of patient acuity and diversity.

This next section offers specific suggestions for playing the game of process group therapy in the PHP/IOP setting. It discusses the posture of the clinician in addition to the strategies of structure and routine, group schedule, the daily assessment/check-in, and relevant group therapy techniques.

The Posture of the Clinician

Prior to using any strategy, the clinician should evaluate his or her personal contribution to the group. The clinician is the one constant in the milieu and should have an understanding of how to shape a process group. He or she is balancing task orientation with empathy.

Part of the suggested task-oriented approach is a clinician demonstrating an attitude of calmness, dignity, discretion, and humility. The clinician would not have a job if not for patients. Clinicians should address patients in a nonparental tone. They should view angry outbursts and the making of threats as immature behavior. They should address such patients calmly with few words.

Clinicians have a dual responsibility with crying patients. Although crying is an intimate expression of emotion, it normally elicits anxiety in others. The clinician has an opportunity to model for the group how to stay calm when someone is crying.[21] The clinician must also give dignity to the crying patient by calmly giving the patient a tissue in a normal speed of movement and either (a) observing a respectful silence while the patient finishes talking or (b) continuing to calmly talk to the crying patient in a normal or slightly softer tone of voice about the issue causing the tears.[22] This empathetic approach balances the clinician's task orientation in both structuring and educating the group.

---

[21] A beginning rubric for staying calm is practicing a modified boredom. This enhances the appearance of the clinician modeling an appearance of control and competence. The patient is crying and will eventually stop crying.

[22] The clinician often has to set limits with other patients trying to engage in caretaking of crying patients. The boundaries should come in the forms of nonverbal hand gestures or minimal verbal prompts. The clinician can also move the group into a discussion about crying as an expression of emotion.

The Strategy of Structure and Routine

Because of the acuity, diversity, and time limits that affect the group, the PHP/IOP group as an open group requires a continuity of structure in the forms of consistent rules and clinician direction. The rules serve as a tool to ensure that the group meets a therapeutic standard. The clinician needs to direct group focus about basic recovery and symptom management. As part of the structure, the group should have a routine schedule and an order. The clinician will likely have more success as the agent of structure within the group by observing continuity in the structural elements.

The number of necessary group rules depends on institutional policy and the cohort. Many agencies and hospitals already have certain rules that must be observed in the program. The organization rules are typically related to state law and accreditation. If there is more than one group being held simultaneously in the program, there should be continuity with all groups using the same set of rules. Adult cohorts should have fewer rules than child and adolescent cohorts, and so the clinician will actually be a proactive agent of structure rather than a reactive enforcer of rules in the adult cohort.[23]

Any change in the rules needs to be unilateral to reduce the likelihood of patient splitting. A group, and possibly the whole, can be disrupted when one staff member in another group institutes a new rule. Given that the milieu is more like an economy than an environment, patients will discuss the differences among the clinicians and make comments or complaints and can instigate drama.

Through both the data collection and the directive approach of group leadership, the clinician aims to create a common and safe experience; the proactive interventions used should amount to a focus on the patient's face-value symptomology. The clinician should make it a priority to initiate a common experience among the group members about occurrences of shared symptomology and individual patient efforts to recover.

As a component of the milieu, a routine schedule is a crucial aspect of group therapy in the PHP/IOP setting. The sessions should begin and end on time, and continuity should be practiced with regard to the different group elements. Order is necessary in managing a group of people to achieve the daily tasks.

---

[23] Actual group rules for adults should be few in number. Having numerous rules for a group of adults can be patronizing, condescending, and not therapeutic.

The Strategy of the Daily Self-Assessment

The daily self-assessment is usually a clinical instrument or worksheet that serves the clinician's purpose in gathering the necessary clinical information. The patient can use the self-assessment to make a subjective report of his or her condition and concerns and can discreetly report suicidal ideations or other needs requiring clinician attention.

The daily assessment form should have several elements:

- The patient's name and date
- Scalar questions by which to measure mood and anxiety and any other desired clinical issue[24]
- Questions about suicidal and homicidal ideation
- Functioning questions about sleep, appetite, and concentration

There has been no identifiable research on a best practice for a daily assessment form; pragmatically, a reasonable standard should be utilization manuals that are used by the organization and/or the pertinent MCOs.

The form should be brief and be written in simple language. It should avoid the use of overt clinical jargon. It should be brief so that a patient struggling with focus and attention can complete it with a minimum of frustration. It needs to be organized such that the clinician can readily scan the suicidal and homicidal ideation questions. Appendix D contains some examples of daily assessment forms.[25]

As part of the task-oriented approach, the daily assessment should be completed by the patient at the beginning of the program day and turned in to the clinician at the beginning of the first group, which will give the clinician a chance to review and act accordingly before the patients leave. The clinician should scan it early in the program hour to determine whether patient follow-up is necessary. The clinician will then combine the contents of daily assessment with the objective observations of the patient's affective state and group participation to compose the clinical service note or documentation.

---

[24] Scales are essentially arbitrary. They can be ascending or descending in form. The key is to communicate sufficiently to the patient the meaning of the values so that the patient demonstrates understanding of that scale.

[25] Some organizations and administrators have preexisting, official patient surveys. A clinician may have no input into the creation or revision of such a form.

When using the daily assessment, it helps to recognize its inherent properties and limits. It is an attempt to quantifiably measure a patient's subjective report on a given day that attempts to use continuous, ordinal, and nominal variables.[26] It is only valid to the extent that:

- The patient is truthful about his or her condition.
- The patient is capable of answering in an intact manner.
- The patient understands the meaning of the scales.

Some patients overstate or understate their true conditions that are incongruent with the clinician's objective observation. Some patients avoid reporting suicidal or homicidal ideations. A patient's inability to answer a daily assessment may be due to illiteracy, insufficient English-language skills, or cognitive impairment due to mental illness or substance use. Without elaboration, the scales on a daily assessment have many validity risks because a patient can be confused about whether a scale is ascending or descending. In the end, the daily assessment form serves as a cue to the clinician whether to address further clinical issues and suggests whether clinical progress is made.

Depending on the chosen content, the daily assessment sheet also can constitute a survey of patient concerns that indicates commonalities, which the clinician can utilize in facilitating group discussions. This survey can be used if none of the patients readily has a desire to talk about personal issues in the group.

Running the PHP/IOP Process Group

This section suggests a strategy for conducting a 2-hour therapy group in the PHP/IOP setting. The game plan includes use of a daily assessment survey, a specific group order, and a set of techniques.

The first stage of the group should be an introduction and a review of the confidentiality disclaimer.[27] Part of the implicit structure of both the

---

[26] A continuous variable can take on any value. An ordinal variable can be ranked. A nominal variable measures whether something simply exists.

[27] A suggested disclaimer is "We will practice confidentiality here in the group, but there is a limit of safety to it. By state law, I am a mandatory reporter in that if someone reports abuse or neglect, I am required to call the protective services. Also, if someone reports thoughts of wanting to hurt or kill someone, I am required to warn the 'someone.' Otherwise what is said here will stay here."

milieu and group is that the clinician is subject to specific laws and policies. After the clinician's disclaimer, the clinician should have patients introduce themselves by first name only to new patients.[28]

The second stage is collection of the daily assessments. The clinician should quickly scan the assessments for suicidal and homicidal ideations while beginning the check-ins.

The third stage of check-ins serves a dual purpose of a group-building and monitoring vehicle. The clinician facilitates the self-disclosure of patients while monitoring patient thought content and affective state. The check-in can be about how the patients are feeling on a particular day and/or about how their evenings were.[29] The clinician should start with a returning patient already oriented to the program who can model how to do the check-in. (If all patients are new admissions, then where the clinician starts is arbitrary.) The clinician will then proceed around the circle and prompt each patient to make a similar report.

The fourth stage is open discussion of patient issues. The clinician can choose several catalyzing approaches:

- Asking the group as a whole if anyone wants to talk
- Taking a list of who wants to talk
- Reviewing out aloud the list of concerns from the daily assessment and anonymously reporting the most common concern among the patients
- Asking a specific discussion question[30]

This is the stage during which the clinician should prompt the group members to interact with each other by giving feedback. The therapist has a risk of conducting individual therapy with each patient instead of catalyzing a group process. When a patient poses a question directly to the clinician, the clinician should scan while deflecting to the group in the form of the question: "What does the group think?"

The clinician should also deflect the energy of a patient whether it is anger or anxiety and make it work in the group. There is a human tendency to seek to pacify a challenging or emotional patient, but the

---

[28] This could be excluded on days when there are no new patients.

[29] The goal is to get patients talking in the check-in stage.

[30] Appropriate questions include "What is working for any of you in getting well? What is not working in getting well?"

clinician can maintain a power position and catalyze group process by asking "Does anyone else relate to this?"

A surprising tool used to deflect patient energy and catalyze group process is silence. Silence is uncomfortable for anxious individuals, and patients will start giggling or someone who cannot tolerate the silence will speak up. The clinician can then lead a productive group discussion on anxiety.

Productive groups in the PHP/IOP setting usually occur when patients disclose their feelings and issues and in turn give feedback to each other. When the group has reached this state of functioning, the clinician has been successful in catalyzing a group process and only has to monitor for redirection and documentation purposes.

Some groups can be unproductive when patients are problem focused and are talking about how helpless they all feel. The clinician may have to prompt patients at times to explore possible solutions.

Whether a group is productive or unproductive, a clinician will often have to act as a timekeeper in the group when a number of patients want time to talk. In such cases, the clinician should say that an effort will be made to give everyone the opportunity to talk. The clinician may have to stop a patient at a subject change and politely say "We need to give others a chance to talk." Whether or not every patient got a chance to talk, it is crucial that the group end at the scheduled time.

When there is time at the end of the group, discharging patients should be allowed a meaningful opportunity to say good-bye. Because of the intimacy and emotional bonds, discharges can engender a sense of grief and loss in both the discharging and remaining patients, which can detract from treatment focus. Practicing a group good-bye ritual can serve several purposes:

- It aids in the recovery of the grief and loss created by the discharge.
- It enhances group quality through the message of hope that patients recover.
- It refocuses patients on treatment and uses the emotional energy as momentum to catalyze group process for the next program day.[31]

---

[31] Processing the good-bye ritual in the group can prompt patients to evaluate what is needed to be successfully discharged. It also could be a springboard to a discussion about grief and loss on the next program day.

If the group members have made emotional good-byes, the clinician can reflect the emotional reactions of the patients as indicators that the group has been a meaningful and helpful therapeutic experience.

Treatment Planning as an Aid to a Successful Group Experience

The weekly treatment planning session can be a tool for encouraging a patient to participate meaningfully in the group. The clinician can use the opportunity to encourage the patient to discuss the most significant stressors when appropriate in the group. As discussed in Chapter 3, a treatment plan goal can be that a patient will talk about his or her primary stresses in the group. The clinician who is both the therapist and case manager can monitor patient progress on this goal.

Some anxious patients try to talk about their issues only to the clinician in one-on-one sessions and, in turn, avoid talking in the group. This avoidance of group participation turns the treatment planning session into an inappropriate individual therapy. The clinician may need to set limits with these patients and redirect them to self-disclose in the group.[32]

SOME COMMON PROBLEMS

This section discusses common group problems that occur in the PHP/IOP setting. All of these problems reflect the reality that the group is a subset of the milieu that includes both staff and patients. The first problem occurs when a new clinician takes over a group. Another problem arises when a patient obsesses about another patient's needs to the point of complaining about the clinician not doing enough. A third problem occurs when a shadow group evolves into a cabal. This section suggests some strategies to use to address these group problems.

The New Clinician

When a new or different clinician takes over a group, there is often dramatic dissatisfaction by patients with personality-disorder traits. These

---

[32] In the United States, Medicare and commercial insurances do not usually pay for individual therapy in adult PHPs/IOPs.

patients are likely exhibiting some level of abandonment by the former clinician. The poor ego functioning of these patients comes out in the form of passive-aggressive drama in which the patients scapegoat the new clinician as a villain with various nebulous and emotional complaints. Some patients triangulate another staff member into the drama by making a threat of physical harm toward the new clinician, leaving the staff member with a duty to warn. The drama resulting during a transition can throw a milieu into a temporary uproar.

Handling this drama requires adherence to standards, staff cooperation, and the support of the new clinician. The staff can manage it by empathetic listening and responding minimally to the emotion. Patient complaints should be scrutinized for any hard facts versus being merely emotional in nature. Limits must be set with patients who make threats of physical aggression toward staff. Complaining patients can be offered discharge or transfer to another group, if available. If the clinician and staff can remain calm and rational, the patient drama will subside.

The Defocusing Patient

Often a patient will defocus from treatment by focusing on another patient's problems. Such a patient will take ownership of the other's problems to the point of worry. Out of the worry, the defocusing patient will instigate drama by complaining to other staff or the supervisor that the clinician is not doing enough.

The suggested approach is to attend to the patient's complaint to defuse the emotion and then encourage him or her to focus on his or her own treatment. The supervisor or the other staff member can deliver this message or refer the complainant back to the clinician to do it. It is crucial for the staff to communicate among themselves about such a matter to avoid staff splitting and undermining of the clinician.

The Cabal

Another form of drama that occurs is a cabal emanating from a shadow group. The shadow group forms from two or more patients who tend to be codependent if not personality disordered. The shadow group forms during the breaks between group therapy hours or outside program hours. It becomes enmeshed due to poor emotional boundaries.[33] The transition to being a cabal occurs when a member of the shadow group acts as spokesperson and complains about the quality of the clinician to another staff member. If one of the cabal personally attacks the clinician, most of the cabal will be absent the next day. The high level of emotion that results from a cabal can defocus the group and detract from the treatment of other patients.

The suggested strategy for dealing with the shadow group/cabal has three parts. When the clinician recognizes that there is an enmeshed shadow group, he or she should increase the directive stance toward the group. The directive stance includes more wheel-spoke patterns of interaction and frequent announcements about the importance of being on time to group sessions. Second, treatment planning sessions should aim to intensify the focus of each of the shadow group members on individual treatment goals.[34] Third, the clinician should advise the other staff members during daily staffing or other informal periods about the appearance of a shadow group or cabal and ask the other staff to refer the matter back to the clinician when possible to avoid staff splitting. The three interventions of this strategy behaviorally shape the focus of the group and the individual patients away from cabal activities.

A common thread of the strategies is staff cooperation. The cooperation does require insight into these problems and a common game plan. If the clinician and staff do not cooperate on addressing these group problems, the problems can escalate and the therapeutic milieu could be disrupted.

---

[33] The shadow group often consists of patients on medical leave or those with disability. These patients sometimes fill their time and distract themselves by getting into the affairs of others.

[34] Refocusing the individual members of the cabal includes discussing how short-term treatment is and that the patient will be discharged soon. The discussion with each patient should be solely on that patient's goals. The clinician should avoid mentioning any of the other patients in the cabal. If the patient brings up the problems of other patients, the clinician may have to remind the patient about why he or she is in treatment.

CONCLUSIONS

This chapter presented the game of process group therapy in the PHP/IOP setting. Group therapy is the standard form of therapy at this level of care as one clinician can simultaneously work with multiple patients. Although not all of the cohorts equally benefit from it, process group therapy has the potential to yield rich benefits to participating patients through the exchange of self-disclosure and feedback.

Process group therapy in the PHP/IOP group has challenges and limits. Groups have patients of various acuity and functioning levels. There is the potential of a high degree of social diversity in a group. The group also tends to have a high turnover of patients. Not all patients will participate to an equal degree for various reasons. In the midst of these challenges, the clinician is a multitasking catalyst leading relative strangers to become a therapy group while simultaneously monitoring their symptomology.

In light of these challenges, the game of running an effective process group in the PHP/IOP setting is one of efficiency, structure, and routine. Having patients complete a daily assessment form before a group session allows the clinician to gather subjective, clinical information efficiently. Following a daily script in which the clinician is a strong leader can rapidly catalyze the formation of a therapeutic group. Using the treatment-planning sessions to coach patients on group participation enhances the likelihood of meaningful therapeutic exchange. Continuity in these three practices tends to increase the therapeutic value of the group experience for each patient.

Some of the recurring group problems exist because the group is a subset of a larger milieu. The program staff must cooperate to manage the problems of group adjustment to a new clinician, a defocusing patient, and a defocusing cabal.

Group process therapy in the PHP/IOP setting can be a daunting challenge for the novice clinician. This chapter has offered some principles toward reducing that challenge into successful and meaningful practice that can help improve the lives of patients.

REFERENCE

Yalom, I., & Leszcz, M. (2005). *The theory and practice of group psychotherapy* (5th ed.). New York, NY: Basic Books.

CHAPTER SEVEN

PSYCHOEDUCATION

Psychoeducation refers to the education given to patients as part of their treatment. It can be about symptoms, medications, treatment in general, coping skills, and lifestyle issues related to recovery. It is considered to be a standard part of the levels of care of both the partial hospitalization program (PHP) and the intensive outpatient program (IOP). Payer sources usually require licensed clinicians to provide psychoeducational services in the PHP/IOP setting.[1]

Through psychoeducation, the clinician and program staff should present patients with useful information that will engender insight or impart skills. The clinician should embrace the role of the confident and knowledgeable professional who has something to offer to patients to help them improve their lives.

The type of psychoeducation needed depends on the cohort. Younger cohorts will benefit more from basic life skills such as hygiene and health. Adult and geriatric cohorts will benefit from abstract and cognitive subjects. The chronic cohort may benefit more from illness management. The depth and length of the educational sessions should vary, based on the ability of the patients to use the information realistically.[2]

Because a PHP/IOP is an economic product provided to the patients, it is in the interest of the program staff to have quality psychoeducation. Although it does not have to be entertaining, it should be interesting, polished, and delivered with some level of genuine passion. A psychoeducational effort should be well organized and coordinated so as to offer patients a variety of relevant topics.

If one or more staff members is lackadaisical and apathetic about presenting psychoeducation, it will detract from the milieu and can

---

[1] This requirement does depend on the payer source and so there are exceptions.

[2] The length of the presentation also varies, based on payer source requirements. Adults may have longer sessions than children and adolescents.

precipitate staff splitting in the form of complaints that rate one clinician as better than the other. When it is done well, psychoeducation enhances the treatment and recovery of patients, increases patient satisfaction, and contributes to a positive therapeutic milieu.

This chapter assumes that the clinician is working with a team of other clinicians in the PHP/IOP unit in a hospital or agency situation rather than as a solo clinician working in a private practice. Although the teamwork aspects will be irrelevant, some of the content on organization and routinization will still be applicable to the solo IOP practitioner.

This chapter discusses the game of psychoeducation in the PHP/IOP setting. It discusses the challenges to imparting psychoeducation at this level of care. It then suggests a game for organizing, implementing, and evaluating a psychoeducational rotation that can be integrated into the existing workload of the clinician.

THE CHALLENGES OF PSYCHOEDUCATION IN THE PHP/IOP SETTING

Although the significance varies from cohort to cohort, the challenges of psychoeducation at the PHP/IOP level are both patient related and staff related. The patient challenges pertain to redundancy and appropriateness to the cohort. The staff challenges are organizing, creating, and maintaining continuity. This section elaborates on these challenges.

The general patient challenges are redundancy, discreteness, and safety. All three challenges relate to the structure of the milieu and the quality of the program.

Redundancy

The challenge of redundancy refers to clinical staff repeating the same educational material to the same group of patients. The redundancy may happen several times within a patient's stay. Redundancy typically occurs when the clinicians do not cooperate on what psychoeducation is presented. Redundancy can cast an unprofessional shadow on the program staff and diminish the quality of the product that is delivered to the patients.

In addition to basic patient dissatisfaction, redundancy can create milieu disruption. If there is a significant presence of patients with personality or impulsive disorders, redundancy can precipitate a negative group contagion. Patients with personality-disorder traits and impulse control disorders are likely to complain that they have heard a subject already. The complaining patients may also engage in staff splitting that includes comparing the presentation skills of clinicians. The risks of redundancy are detraction from treatment focus and possible premature discharges.

Redundancy is also a symptom of the clinical staff not appreciating the value of continuity in treatment. Some of the lack of demonstrated appreciation may be due to a negative personality trait of one or more of the staff, or it could be a matter of personality conflict. Because staff relationships and interactions are a structural component of the milieu, if the staff members do not cooperate in the delivery of psychoeducation, the quality of the milieu is degraded and it is at risk for chaos. Supervisory or management intervention may be required if there are personality-based impediments to coordinated psychoeducation.

Discreteness

The challenge of discreteness refers to the separateness of each psychoeducational presentation. For a psychoeducational presentation to be discrete, it should stand alone and give patients a complete summary of the salient or relevant points on the issue or skill. Discreteness also implies that a clinician is neither referring to previous psychoeducational presentations nor talking about upcoming educations. A discrete presentation is not a continuation or the second part of a previous program day's presentation, nor will it continue into the next program day.

Discreteness is an important aspect of program quality in situations with higher patient acuity and high patient turnover. Discreteness is a subtle, punctilious element that enhances the sense of order in a milieu structure. The patients are not necessarily going to recognize it when it is present, but some problems may arise when it is not practiced.

The problems related to the absence of discreteness are relatively small, but given the intensity of the PHP/IOP setting, they can accumulate with other milieu factors and evolve into significant milieu disruption. First, new admissions and patients who are being discharged are deprived of beneficial information from the missed portion. A two-part presentation may also be too long and detailed for the attention span of patients with acuity. Third, patients with personality-disorder traits may be unable to cope with the suspense of having to wait for the second part or having missed the first part and will be more likely to engage in related drama that agitates the milieu.[3] Clinicians may have to spend extra time with patients in these cases, either pacifying or going over the information privately with them, which adds to a clinician's workload.[4]

The patient challenge of safety refers to the avoidance of overly provocative trauma-related subjects. Although there is the likelihood of a high comorbidity of posttraumatic stress disorder (PTSD) among the patients in a PHP/IOP at any one time,[5] the acuity of such patients reduces their capability of coping through the retraumatizing that comes with such discussion. A patient with greater acuity has a greater risk of being overwhelmed by the dissociative nature of flashbacks to the point of developing suicidal ideations and needing inpatient hospitalization. The reality is that the PHP/IOP setting is a risky setting to make trauma a regular psychoeducational topic.[6]

The staff challenges to psychoeducation at the PHP/IOP level of care center around cooperation. It will take staff cooperation to plan, organize, and maintain a psychoeducational program that is safe, has discrete presentations, and avoids redundancy. Barring the subject of

---

[3] The personality-disordered patient may be stressed by the suspense if aware of the schedule of presentations. One other milieu distraction related to a personality-disordered patient disrupting a milieu with drama is when a patient strongly verbalizes how important an upcoming education presentation is and then he or she is absent on the day of that presentation. In this second scenario, the patient is engaging in self-sabotage or self-victimization.

[4] If this does happen, it is indicative of a number of staff problems, including a staff member with control issues who does not appreciate that the order in a milieu is a cooperative venture.

[5] See Kessler et al. (1995).

[6] The milieu can be degraded by a large number of rehospitalizations. New patients who are significantly anxious and have problems with rational thinking may see the frequent migration to inpatient care and either leave the treatment or go to a competing program. Patients do notice whether other patients in a program are improving.

trauma, the actual topics selected are secondary to staff agreement on the topics.[7] Although the subjects presented are important, the level of staff cooperation has a far greater bearing on the therapeutic milieu. Given the intense environment of the milieu and the assumption that more than one clinician is sharing the psychoeducational duties in addition to other job responsibilities, it will eventually be evident if staff cooperation does not exist as evidenced by milieu disruptions.

Staff identification of psychoeducational subjects presents another challenge. The psychoeducational efforts are elements of the milieu structure that the staff is creating. Staff members will need to agree on what subjects should be presented and who will present them. This process will be either a staff-building exercise or a source of staff conflict.

After the subjects have been identified, staff members are often challenged with creating or locating appropriate materials. Commercially prepared material is often cost prohibitive and becomes outdated sooner than expected.[8] Video materials especially can wear out over time and lose the appearance of relevance with outdated slang, clothing, and hairstyles. Furthermore, copyrighted materials cannot be photocopied unless they are in the public domain. The reality is that the PHP/IOP staff will have to create presentations and materials and develop those presentations in addition to agreeing on rotating schedules for presenting them.

THE GAME OF PSYCHOEDUCATION

The suggested game is a psychoeducational rotation for the PHP/IOP setting. The game applies more to adult cohorts than to children and adolescents, but the strategy can be generalized to programs serving the younger patient populations. The ideal outcome of the game is the production and maintenance of a quality psychoeducational routine or rotation that avoids redundancy, practices discreteness, and enables clinicians to be efficient and effective in their other work duties.

---

[7] This chapter avoids suggesting what subjects should be chosen. The important matter is that the clinician and relevant staff agree on what should be presented.

[8] There tends to be more published material available for children and adolescents than for adults.

The first stage of the game involves evaluation and planning. The relevant clinicians should evaluate the average length of stay in a program and the patient's educational needs. Identifying a number of discrete educational topics may be a matter of brainstorming.

A worksheet in the form of a calendar grid should be created and used to enter the educational topics. Thematic weeks could be created as long as the topics are discrete. Figure 7.1 is an example of an educational rotation.

Negotiation is a part of the rotation's organization process. The clinicians should negotiate the subjects they will present and the days on which they will present them.[9] An important consideration in this negotiation is that clinicians with strengths or expertise in certain areas should present those subjects. The spirit of the negotiation should seek to balance clinician satisfaction and interest with the understanding that cooperation is necessary for the development and maintenance of the PHP/IOP milieu.[10]

	Monday (Bob)	Tuesday (Cecily)	Wednesday (Bob)	Thursday (Arthur)	Friday (Francis)
Week #1	Boundaries	Family dysfunction	Codependency	Grief and loss	Developing social relationships
Week #2	Self-care	Self-esteem	Self-control	Understanding 12 programs in recovery	Feelings
Week #3	Anger management	Anxiety management	Understanding depression	Meaning and significance	Time management
Week #4	Fair fighting	Assertiveness	Self-talk	Workplace coping	Relaxation skills

Figure 7.1 *An example of a psychoeducational rotation.*

---

[9] A good negotiation tool is offering hesitant clinicians the first choice on the subjects and days they wish to present. Another good tool is allowing the hesitant clinicians to use the existing materials.

[10] Some supervisors may choose to organize the rotation and assign the topics, but given that master's-level clinicians are highly motivated professionals, staff morale will likely be improved if they can have ownership. Ownership increases the intrinsic value of the work and encourages fidelity to maintaining the milieu.

A department or agency may already have some suitable materials for some of the educational topics that clinicians can use. Given that clinicians are likely to already be busy with other duties, these materials should be used to accelerate the implementation of rotation.[11]

Beyond the existing educational materials, sources for other educational subjects will likely be available in books or on the Internet. The Internet offers an advantage in that the clinician can copy and paste text and some graphics into word-processing or publishing software and easily shape this into psychoeducational material. There are many convenient Internet websites that provide useful materials that can be adapted to a clinician's preference.

There are three caveats regarding Internet materials. First, many materials are copyrighted and cannot be photocopied and distributed to patients. Although there is a lot of free material on the Internet, the clinician should consider the website's credibility, as anyone can create a website. Finally, the Internet is dynamic, and websites come and go and are revised, and material can disappear. Given the caveats, a clinician should consider adapting or integrating Internet-derived materials into originally created presentations.[12,13]

Patient handouts add value to psychoeducational presentations. Patients with acute symptoms may not have their normal levels of comprehension and memory and can benefit from having the handouts to review at a later date.[14] In light of likely patient acuity, handouts should be brief with bullet points as opposed to large portions of text. Furthermore,

---

[11] Pragmatically, the existing materials should be presented in the earlier weeks of the first time through the rotation so that clinicians have time to create the materials for the later subjects in the rotation.

[12] A clarifying question for evaluating a website for use in an educational presentation is whether it is mainstream information.

[13] Notwithstanding the caveats about the Internet, a good website for materials is http://coping.us/ (used with the permission of James Messina, PhD). Overall, the most dependable Internet sources for psychoeducational materials are government agency websites. There are a number of U.S. and Canadian government-related websites with credible and adaptable materials that are in the public domain.

[14] Adults tend to be larger consumers of handouts. Children and adolescents tend to ascribe little value to handouts.

the handouts should guide patients as to how to apply the subject matter to their situations.

As part of the milieu and team-building processes, clinicians should review and critique each other's presentations and handouts. This peer review serves several purposes:

- Clinicians can give each other advice on the practicality and validity of the material.
- Because they are familiar with the material, clinicians can substitute for each other when on vacation and on sick leave, thus maintaining program continuity.
- Staff agreement on the material reduces the likelihood of patient–staff splitting and minimizes the drama that may be instigated by some of the more sensitive personality-disordered patients who complain about being offended by the subject matter.[15]

When the psychoeducational materials have been assembled, they should be kept in a central location for access. Hard copies of the rotation, presentation outlines, and handout originals should be kept in a centralized notebook.[16] A sufficient supply of copies of each handout could be kept in a central file for ready access. Depending on the technology resources available to the department, PDF files of all presentations and handouts could be kept on a central drive or server for easy printing and reduction of clutter. To maintain continuity in the rotation, digital storage is preferable for efficiency, but hard copies of the handouts should be kept as backup in case computers or servers are down.

A rotation should be coordinated by the use of a centrally visible calendar. The day of the rotation should be marked on the designated day. Clinicians should be able to look at the calendar and see whether it is their turn in the rotation. When a program is closed for holidays or inclement weather, the missed psychoeducational sessions should not be

---

[15] Some examples of this splitting are (a) antisocial personalities complaining about an anger management presentation, and (b) patients claiming to be embarrassed for other patients in the room.

[16] For accreditation purposes, the information may need to be incorporated in a program plan. Furthermore, because technology can fail, having hard-copy originals allows program staff to maintain continuity.

made up because this would disturb the rotation, which is a punctilious element of the therapeutic milieu.

After one or two passes through the rotation, the staff and supervisor should evaluate rotation performance. Staff should make mutually agreed-upon changes or adjustments to the rotation, which fit the needs of the patients and the workloads of the clinicians. Staff should not hesitate to change or polish a psychoeducational rotation if all agree that it is necessary for effectiveness, efficiency, the needs of patients, and the structure of the therapeutic milieu.

As the staff repeats the rotation, the quality of the presentation and execution should improve. Clinicians will likely refine their presentations and the rotation becomes part of the clinician's work routine.

When a new clinician joins a team, it is important for the milieu and for continuity that a renegotiation takes place. Although the new clinician should work to fit within the staff, the staff should assist him or her to acclimate as soon as possible to minimize inherent disruptions to the milieu and to achieve a new routine.

CONCLUSIONS

This chapter suggested a game for organizing, implementing, and evaluating a psychoeducational strategy in the PHP/IOP setting that both undergirds the therapeutic milieu and can be integrated into the existing workload of the clinician. Psychoeducation is an expected element of the PHP/IOP for payer sources, and if it is unorganized, there is the risk that the disorganization itself will precipitate milieu disruption or intensify the existing chaos, which detracts from treatment focus. An orderly and well-executed psychoeducational program enhances milieu structure and creates positive economic externalities that include greater patient satisfaction and higher attendance.

The development of the psychoeducational strategy requires staff cooperation in the evaluation, planning, and implementation phases. Although the psychoeducational topics should avoid overtly provocative subjects, the greater matter is that the staff is in agreement and works together to produce and implement the rotation. Staff cooperation is at the heart of a milieu's structure and stability.

One objection or counterpoint to the strategy of a psychoeducational rotation in the PHP/IOP setting is that it is rigid and does not allow opportunity for staff to meet the needs of individual patients. This objection is valid to the point that there will be patient diversity, which includes needing information and coping skills that are not part of the rotation. However, because the focus in the PHP/IOP setting is the stabilization of patients in groups, such unique patient needs will not be addressed nor must they be imminently addressed in the psychoeducational rotation. The rotation is an efficiency and structural approach that allows for meeting the needs of the maximum patients at one time while allowing the clinician to address any unique patient needs in individual treatment planning or case management sessions.

CHAPTER EIGHT

SAFETY ISSUES

As a gathering point for human beings who are in distress, the partial hospitalization program (PHP)/intensive outpatient program (IOP) setting is connected with violence, danger, and abuse. Patients have often previously experienced violence and abuse. They may have been or currently are in danger and may be dangerous to themselves and others. Patients will report this information, and the clinicians and PHP/IOP staff constantly have to evaluate whether the information requires action in view of safety.

For the purposes of this chapter, *safety* means reducing the risk of harm to patients or other relevant individuals in accordance with any such applicable laws and professional ethical imperatives. Safety can also mean risk reduction for the clinician and the program staff.

Safety, liability, and risk management for the helping professions have long been matters of concern and intense focus. Every U.S. state and Canadian province has regulatory bodies tasked with ensuring that the public is safe and not in danger when in treatment. Such regulatory bodies often review complaints that professionals were neglectful of patient safety needs. As part of accreditation standards and legal advice, hospitals and agencies have detailed safety policies and procedures and risk management personnel whose job it is to investigate allegations and incidents.[1]

The typical PHP/IOP in a hospital setting will likely be subject to the existing organizational infrastructure and policy.[2] The employee of such a program (whether clinical or nonclinical) is typically given initial orientation and then is responsible for maintaining awareness of and compliance with the relevant laws and policies.

---

[1] The Joint Commission has a policy of publicizing a wide variety of safety goals that include suicide prevention in the hospital setting.

[2] Some policies are not necessarily in the policy manuals but can consist of verbal direction or memos from supervisors and administrators.

Nevertheless, the PHP/IOP clinician still has to practice oversight in patient safety as the line-level professional who is directly observing patient behavior and receiving information. A clinician may get a call from a family member that the patient is making suicidal comments outside of the program hours, while making no such disclosure in the program. The PHP/IOP clinician and staff may receive second-hand information that a patient has been abusive or has made homicidal threats outside of the program. A patient may disclose having been abusive to a child or spouse. A spouse may report that a patient is threatening him or her. In dealing with safety incidents and handling allegations, it is possible that the clinician and the department will be thoroughly scrutinized by the organization's risk management team and government inspectors.[3]

This chapter reviews the concerns of safety and risk management in the PHP/IOP. It elaborates on ways of making the milieu safe. It discusses suicidal and aggressive patients. It explains how to gracefully play the game of having to make a protective services report and maintain relationships with the patients and/or their families. Finally, it analyzes safety issues pertaining to sex, trauma, religion, politics, and confidentiality.

SAFETY CHALLENGES

Challenges to safety in the PHP/IOP setting must be considered within the context of the clinician's intense workpace and the multiple demands he or she faces. A clinician must be mindful of the patient's clinical presentation because patient emergencies often occur at inconvenient times for the clinician. A clinician must be flexible enough to change focus and activity immediately when a patient crisis situation occurs.

Clinicians also face a challenge of countertransference in potentially dangerous situations. In all of their hostility and dramatic unpleasantness, difficult patients verbalize suicidal comments in both direct and passive-aggressive manners. Difficult adult patients may also report they have hit their children, but portray themselves as victims in the process. Difficult patients may act entitled as a motivation for being abusive to other

---

[3] The private practice IOP may not have the detailed risk management policy.

patients in the program. As a human, the clinician has to compartmentalize natural, negative emotions and maintain an objective perspective and presentation when difficult patients manifest dangerous behaviors.

The Challenges of Suicidal Patients

A suicidal patient as experienced in the PHP/IOP setting comes in at least two general varieties: one who is gamey (playing games) and one who is straightforward in reporting his or her suicidality. A straightforward patient manifests no particular agenda and is open and seeking when making disclosures about suicidal ideation and any such plan to act on the thoughts. A gamey patient demonstrates a control agenda by not being forthcoming, but instead disclosing suicide attempts a few days after the so-called attempts, which precludes the criteria for admission as an inpatient.[4] Furthermore, the gamey patient may actually engage in a suicide attempt by overdose on the program site. Although staff members want to be on top of all clinical situations, including suicidal patients, this requires patient cooperation.

Some gamey patients will send a mixed message of suicidality. A patient may deny suicidality on a checkout survey and then verbalize suicidality to a different staff member. In these cases, the checkout survey is null and void and the patient is sent for reassessment or is hospitalized.

On the other hand, some gamey patients verbalize suicidal ideation, and when referred to the admitting or assessment department, the patient is no longer suicidal at the time of the assessment. The patient may report being suicidal with an inability to contract for safety to the PHP/IOP. The patient then contracts for safety with the assessment clinician. In some cases, this situation repeats itself again and again, because the patient wants to act in such a manner.

----

[4] Two examples of this scenario are (a) a patient reporting on a Tuesday that he or she had overdosed 3 days before on Saturday and (b) a patient reporting that he or she was suicidal with a plan 3 days ago. Both of these scenarios fall outside of the parameters of utilization criteria for inpatient admission. Sometimes these admissions are made in an emotional or dramatic fashion during the group session or to someone else other than the clinician.

The Challenges of Aggressive Patients

The aggressive patient may be verbally threatening or actually physically aggressive. Patients in the younger cohorts are the ones who tend to be physically aggressive, whereas the adult cohorts tend to be at best threatening physical aggression without follow-through.

The child and adolescent cohorts overall have a significant presence of aggressive patients. The patients can be both verbally and physically aggressive toward other patients and toward staff. Younger children, age 9 and younger, typically have physical tantrums because they lack the cognitive development to verbalize feelings and use abstract coping skills. Typically, aggressive adolescent patients are impulsive and do not give a warning if and when they are going to hit someone. Older aggressive children and adolescents may also have lower intellectual functioning in addition to having attention deficit and substance use issues. At times, the PHP/IOP setting may have chaotic milieus dominated by a high prevalence of aggressive children and adolescents who are not treatment focused.

Typically, the aggressive patients in the adult cohort are rare. The aggressive patient is more passive-aggressive than aggressive and actually instigates drama among staff. An aggressive adult patient tends to report to one staff member having homicidal ideation toward another staff member. Given the duty to warn, the informed staff member will tell the threatened staff member about the patient's homicidal ideation toward him or her and a dramatic tension will occur.

Given the likelihood of severe symptoms combined with medication noncompliance, there is a somewhat greater likelihood of aggression in the chronically mentally ill cohort. The aggression may arise out of either psychosis or mood issues. This particular cohort does have patients who can get physically aggressive, but typically, the disruptive behavior tends most often to consist of verbal outbursts.

THE GAME OF SAFETY

The game of safety is a principled and philosophical game that is intertwined with basic milieu management. It is about following accepted standards in the handling of situations. Safety practices must consider order and an appreciation of the inherent limits. Although handling safety issues is stressful and emotionally draining, the professional is expected to have a plan and display calmness when dangerous situations arise. This section discusses some suggested plans or games for safety as a response to the challenges.

The Game of Dealing With the Suicidal Patient

The challenge of the suicidal patient can be complicated as the typical question on most check-in and checkout surveys is "Any thoughts of suicide?" This is vague because there are different levels of suicidality. Some departments and agencies have detailed policies that a patient will be automatically reassessed by the admitting department, whereas others will require the completion of a safety plan. Regardless of whether there is a policy, the onus is on the clinician to interpret the situation and to take the appropriate action.

The principle that a clinician should follow is "the standard of care." This is a standard by which clinical decisions will be judged by the legal system. For all practical purposes, the clinician should follow all organizational policies, and the clinician should discuss the situation with other clinical staff and the patient's psychiatrist or the medical director. The clinician should not act alone in such situations unless it is a clear-cut situation in which the patient meets the criteria for inpatient admission.

A clinician must do a follow-up interview with the suicidal patient to assess for safety. The immediate concern is whether the suicidal patient presents as safe enough to be left alone and out of *eye view*.[5] The second concern is whether the patient is safe enough to leave the program site. Such an interview should include the following questions:

- You indicated that you were having thoughts of suicide. What kind of thoughts are you having?
- When have you been having these thoughts?
- How frequent are these thoughts?

---

[5] Eye view is the practice of not letting a patient leave the sight of a clinician or staff member.

- Have you been thinking of a "plan" as to how you would hurt or kill yourself?[6]
- Do you think that you will be safe if you leave here? Can you contract for safety?

A clinician should initially use the utilization review policy of the agency or hospital as a guiding framework in interpreting interview results.

A typical utilization review policy lays out examples that meet the criteria for an inpatient admission. Typically, a patient meeting the criteria for inpatient admission due to suicidality will be an immediate safety risk, which includes (a) suicidal ideation with a plan, (b) suicidal ideation with an inability to contract for safety, and (c) command hallucinations telling a patient to kill himself. If there is any vagueness in the patient's answers or if a patient seems to be playing games with the answers, the patient's psychiatrist should be consulted. Where there is no psychiatrist as in the cases of commercial insurance IOP, the medical director should be consulted and the patient should be referred back to the admitting department for reassessment.[7]

If the patient reports having active thoughts about suicide, the clinician should make an immediate check for pills or sharp objects. There should be no assumption that a patient at the program site is safe. A patient should be asked about having dangerous objects and the clinician should secure any pills or possible sharp objects. If necessary, the clinician should enlist the assistance of other staff members to keep the patient in eye view until the patient is transferred either to the admitting department or to the inpatient unit.

If the patient is actively reporting suicidal thinking with a plan and will not agree to be reassessed, the patient should be placed under a hold or commitment in which he or she is admitted against his or her will. There is significant variance in local and state/provincial policy when it

---

[6] Plans can include overdose of pills or drugs, cutting wrists, using a firearm to shoot self, walking out into traffic, crashing one's car, or jumping off a bridge.

[7] Some hospitals have policies that indicate that a PHP/IOP patient can be directly admitted as an inpatient.

comes to admitting a patient against his or her will.[8] A clinician may have to discuss this option with the gamey patient as an illusion of a choice.[9]

In situations with less than a definitive need for hospitalization, the clinician should err on the side of safety. If the patient presents as being gamey with details or an uncertainty as to whether or not the patient can contract for safety, he or she should be referred to the admitting department for reassessment. A patient having persistent and recurring thoughts of suicide should also be referred to the admitting department for reassessment.[10] The patient having only occasional thoughts of suicide without a plan, who can contract for safety, should complete a safety plan.

Some organizations already have a safety contract form or document as part of their policy. The clinician should use that form as part of the policy. If there is no official safety plan form or policy, the clinician should create a safety plan document as follows:

- The schedule for the remainder of the patient's day
  - How will the patient spend his or her time?
  - What can the patient do differently to distract him or her for the night?
- Person who can be called now to enlist help in keeping the patient safe
  - Can the patient stay with someone who can keep an eye on the patient?
  - Who will take charge of the patient's medicine so as to reduce the likelihood of a temptation to overdose?
  - Who can take any firearms/weapons and secure them?

---

[8] In some localities, a psychiatrist or physician has the authority to place a patient under a time-limited hold. In other localities, a judge must issue a court order for a patient to be admitted against his or her will. Some localities have options both for a physician's order and for a judge's order.

[9] The illusion of choice gives the patient the opportunity to choose to be admitted. The clinician says to the patient, "You can choose to go get reassessed or I will have to have you placed on a hold." A clinician should evaluate what the options are as part of the orientation to the job.

[10] The reassessment by the admitting department is an opportunity to clarify whether the patient is actually safe or whether the patient divulges more information that solidifies a clinical decision to admit the patient as an inpatient.

- The assurance that the patient indicates he or she will return to the program on the next program day
- Documentation of the crisis number of the organization or hospital

The clinician should have the patient sign the document, and the clinician should sign the document. The clinician should then contact the psychiatrist for clearance and contact the designated family member(s) or support person(s). A copy of the safety plan should be placed in the medical record.

The safety plan is predicated on the availability of a patient support system and that the patient has been truthful about his or her situation. If the patient has no support individuals available, the clinician should consult the psychiatrist about whether the patient should be hospitalized anyway, because there is no support system to ensure the patient's safety.

A clinician should document that phone calls were placed to the support persons. When possible, the clinician should have follow-up documentation that the safety measures (medications and weapons are secured) were completed. The documentation should be explicit during phone calls with the psychiatrist and the support persons. Names and phone numbers of the support persons should also be included in the documentation.

If a patient completes a safety plan but does not come back the next day and does not answer the phone, the clinician should contact the patient's support person. If the support person is not available or cannot vouch for the patient's safety, the clinician should call for law enforcement to do a welfare check on the patient.

The disclaimer about a safety plan is that it does not guarantee the patient's safety. The safety plan is an expression of clinical judgment on the part of the clinician and the treatment team that the patient expressing suicidal ideation was safe enough to leave and was cognitively intact to commit to safety. Patients may make a safety plan and still either attempt or commit suicide. If the patient does attempt or commit suicide, the execution of the policy and the safety plan will likely be investigated by the organization regarding what could have been done to avoid the incident. The hope is that the clinician and treatment team acted impeccably according to policy and in good clinical judgment within the standard of care.

The Game of Dealing With the Aggressive Patient

There are three particular situations involving aggressive patients that a clinician and treatment team tend to encounter: (a) the patient threatening the staff, (b) the patient being aggressive toward another patient, and (c) a patient threatening a third person outside of the program or hospital. The agency or hospital may have a set policy to follow in these cases, and the clinician should follow policy when applicable. When no policy exists, the three different situations require different approaches from the clinician and staff.

The situation of the aggressive patient threatening the staff should be handled in a direct manner. As noted earlier, the threatening patient will usually express a desire to a third staff member to hit the targeted staff member. The staff member at the receiving end of the information should inform the targeted staff member. The staff member should first assess the severity of the threat and consult with the psychiatrist as soon as possible whether the patient is in need of hospitalization. As part of the assessment, the staff member should examine whether the patient is mindful of the potential consequences on following through with the threat. Where possible, the patient should be informed of any policy regarding patient aggression toward staff.[11]

When a patient physically acts out toward a clinician or staff member, a crisis situation has occurred. The aggressive patient should then be hospitalized or discharged according to the policy. If a policy does not exist for such situations, pertinent clinical administrators should be immediately called to make a decision about whether the patient should stay in the program.[12]

A patient acting aggressively toward another patient should be handled in much the same way as aggression toward a staff member. The patient who is threatening another patient may need to be discharged or assertively confronted about the potential consequences. The threatened

---

[11] Some hospitals or facilities do not believe in pressing charges against aggressive patients. A clinician should review the organizational policy for this situation. It is often up to an individual clinician to press charges against an aggressive patient.

[12] In the interest of milieu safety, the aggressive patient should be discharged or hospitalized. A patient who hits staff members is too dangerous to stay in a partial program. A 72-hour hold or commitment should be considered.

patient also needs to be informed unless the threats were directly made. A patient who attacks another patient should be admitted to inpatient care as an immediate safety risk. It will be up to the patient and/or patient's guardian whether charges will be pressed against the other patient.[13]

The patient expressing homicidal ideation or threats of aggression toward a third person outside of the program invokes a "duty to warn." In the United States, the duty to warn is mandated by state law in the majority of the states. Most organizations have a defined policy for executing a duty to warn. Law enforcement agencies also have set procedures in place for duty-to-warn reports.[14] In the absence of such a policy, a clinician receiving the report typically needs to notify the threatened individual(s) and the pertinent law enforcement in the jurisdiction where the threatened person lives.

One last situation of aggressiveness occurs when a patient makes an allegation of aggression by a patient or staff member. This patient situation is typically addressed in agency policy as a risk management issue in which designated personnel will conduct an appropriate investigation.

The Protective Services Report

The protective services report presents a delicate situation in which the patient reports having been either the victim or the perpetrator of abuse. The clinician will encounter the need to report when:

- A child or adolescent patient reports being a victim of abuse.
- An adult patient reports that he or she has engaged in domestic violence.
- A family member reports that the patient is being aggressive.
- A patient admits having hit or abused a child or spouse.

---

[13] This situation tends to happen in the child/adolescent cohort but not in the adult cohort. The adult patient who is threatening another patient should be discharged. The child or adolescent making a threat should stay in the program, but if the child or adolescent patient actually hits another patient, he or she should be discharged from the PHP/IOP and admitted as an inpatient.

[14] Some law enforcement agencies may refuse to take the "duty-to-warn" report unless a patient is being admitted to the hospital. Such refusal should be documented in the medical record.

Typically, the clinician is mandated under law to make a report to the pertinent government agency, and a clinician can face various legal consequences and financial liabilities if a report is not made. Given the proliferation of state laws, the average organization tends to have a reporting policy that reflects the law.

Many clinicians will make the report to protective services without telling the patient, but this is risky in that the patient could return and claim victimhood because confidentiality was broken. Depending on the group composition, such a claim of victimhood could paint the clinician as an untrustworthy villain who violated confidentiality and trust, which leads to a chilling effect among the patient population and possibly multiple discharges. Therefore, the clinician has the challenge of making the report while maintaining relationships with the patients and/or their families.

The clinician may have a dilemma when a spouse or partner calls and claims that the patient is being aggressive or threatening at home. The clinician is often in a double bind about discussing such an allegation with the patient because there may not be an official release of information for the clinician to talk with the spouse. This amounts to be a drama situation, where the clinician is being sought as a rescuer by the spouse claiming to be a victim who alleges that the patient is a perpetrator. In terms of good professional boundaries, the clinician cannot act as a police officer in such a case, and out of principle, the clinician should eschew the drama by documenting the spouse's phone call and making a protective services report.

A clinician who must make protective reports may struggle with anxiety and guilt over making reports as it is a reality that some patients will not return for treatment when informed that a protective services or duty-to-warn report must be made. As already noted, many patients may convincingly claim victimhood when a report is made. Nevertheless, a clinician in a PHP/IOP setting will likely have to make many reports over time, and developing a routine for such situations will enhance the likelihood of complying with the law and keeping the patient in treatment.

The routine of dealing with the report starts with the disclaimer. It is a helpful habit to initiate each therapy group and admission with a disclaimer of the reporting requirements. The following is an example of such a disclaimer:

> We will practice confidentiality in the group, but if someone reports abuse or neglect or a threat to hurt someone, I am required by law to make a report to the protective services or the threatened person.

Otherwise what is said here will stay here.

When a patient makes a disclosure in the group, the clinician should privately approach the patient immediately at the end of the session.[15] Confronting the patient in front of the group during a session could cause a preventable chilling effect.

The clinician's routine approach to the patient (whether adult or child) should be low key, calm, humble, and polite. The clinician should frame the discussion because he or she has a requirement to follow the law; this is nothing personal. The clinician should get the pertinent details, such as the time and place of the event and the name and age of the other person involved. In the cases of adults disclosing perpetrated abuse, the clinician often has to use the illusion of choice that the clinician can make the call or the patient can make the call to protective services.

When a child or adolescent discloses that a parent or another family member is the perpetrator of abuse, the clinician should get the information and make the phone call. If the patient claims abuse by a parent who is participating in treatment, the clinician should consider informing the parent face to face at the next available opportunity about having had to make the report in accordance with all laws.[16] The manner of informing that a protective service report was made should also be done in a humble but polite manner with the intent not to hide information from the parents.[17]

If the patient does not return for treatment after the report is made, the clinician should make an amendment to the original report. The amendment should include the information that the patient did not return for treatment after the report and document it in the medical

---

[15] It is possible that some patients make allegations to create an opportunity to disrupt treatment.

[16] Even with stringent reporting laws, the responsible government agency may not act on reports, and the clinician's notice may be the first the parents have heard. Depending on the time lapse between the report and the family session, it may be evident that the responsible agency is not taking action.

[17] This act of informing parental figures of the report can be a power move by the clinician. Such power comes from the strength of character of the clinician. This act of informing also reduces the likelihood that the child or adolescent is merely trying to split the parent(s) and draw the clinician into family drama.

record. It will be up to protective services to render a decision as to what is necessary, as the clinician's responsibility to safety will have ended.

Unsafe Subjects (Sex, Religion, and Politics)

There are a number of subjects that are dangerous to discuss in the PHP/IOP setting—whether in treatment planning or the group. These subjects include sex and sexually related issues, religion, and politics.[18] Discussing these subjects is inevitable, as a few patients will bring them up with the intention of distracting the group process or out of sincere interest. Other patients may cause resulting drama because the subjects get brought up. Some patients bring up the topic and start related drama regarding the discussion. Regardless, patient allegations of staff misconduct involving these subjects can create significant risk problems for the clinician that could include litigation, an internal investigation, termination, a government investigation, and licensure complaints.[19]

The clinician should craft a particular stance that consists of a number of commitments regarding these issues. These commitments include the following:

- The clinician should avoid bringing up risky topics, and when patients bring up those topics (especially the topic of sex), the clinician should discuss the situation with the treatment team members, such as the psychiatrist and nurse.[20]
- The clinician will thoroughly document any such conversations or patient encounters that involve these controversial topics.

---

[18] Existentially, any subject could be a controversial topic for a patient.

[19] A patient can start a conversation about sexual issues and then make allegations that put words in a clinician's mouth. The patient may attempt to cross boundaries by asking a clinician intimate questions. The investigation may produce no conclusive evidence that misconduct occurred but may lead to a notation on the clinician's personnel record, state file, or malpractice insurance account.

[20] If the clinician must bring up the controversial topics, they should relate to the presenting problems on the admission assessment document. The documentation should make a clear connection to the presenting problems.

- The clinician should consider only meeting in rooms with a video monitor, open doors, or large windows where the clinician and patient can be viewed.
- If a sexualized patient wants to talk about sex with a clinician of the opposite sex, it is prudent to refer the patient to a clinician of the same sex.
- When patients bring up the topics in the group, the clinician should consider intervening and setting ground rules regarding the discussion of the topics.[21]

Such ground rules should include that the discussion should be respectful of others with different opinions and that the clinician reserves the right to stop the discussion in the interest of safety.

CONCLUSIONS

This chapter reviewed safety and risk management issues in the PHP/IOP setting and elaborated on making the milieu safe. Dealing with suicidal and aggressive patients should be expected, and principled plans should be developed when there is an absence of official policy. Making a protective services report is a delicate matter that can mean some patients will not return for treatment, but it can be handled in a sensitive way that maintains the therapeutic relationships with patients and/or their families. Sex, religion, and politics are risky subjects that patients will occasionally bring up that should be handled in a straightforward manner but, to minimize risk, should not be dwelled on.

Although it is a rewarding practice setting, a PHP/IOP is an inherently risky therapeutic milieu that requires principled order and thoughtfulness in how safety issues are handled. As reviewed in earlier chapters, it is a potentially volatile milieu where patients with different levels of

---

[21] When it comes to adolescent patients wanting to discuss sex in a group, a clinician's script could include the following: "We can discuss this topic but we must have some ground rules such as (a) This is an embarrassing subject for many so we must be mature, (b) we will not laugh when someone is talking about a personal issue, and (c) I reserve the right to stop the discussion if someone appears to be hurt."

acuity and functioning are assembled for the purpose of treatment. How the clinician and treatment team handle these safety situations either enhances or diminishes the therapeutic nature of the milieu. The clinician and treatment team are expected to be knowledgeable professionals who can handle pertinent crisis situations while maintaining composure.

The beginning clinician will follow an experiential learning curve when handling a particular safety situation in the PHP/IOP setting. It is advisable to debrief with a supervisor and/or colleague about how a situation was handled and what could have been done differently or better. Successful experience and affirmation in handling safety issues does bring about clinician confidence.

Even with confidence and experience in handling safety risks, many clinicians still have angst and anxiety over the potential liabilities in the PHP/IOP setting. To foster peace of mind, a clinician experiencing angst over potential liability should consider purchasing a personal professional liability insurance policy as a supplement to whatever coverage the employer provides.

CHAPTER NINE

THE REGULAR ADULT COHORT

The adult partial hospitalization program (PHP)/intensive outpatient program (IOP) setting serves adults aged 18 to 65 who are of a fairly high functioning level. This group of adult patients is considered to be the "worried well." The patients are mature; have appropriate social skills; and are capable of handling intense, insight-oriented therapy. The program typically serves adults with mood and anxiety disorders. The patients are either step-downs from inpatient care or direct admissions from the community. Patients in this cohort are adults who typically work full time, go to school full time, or are at least not on disability for mental illness.

Because the majority of patients in the cohort are working and have commercial insurance, the managed care organizations (MCOs) are a hegemonic influence in monitoring the patient's condition and clinical decision making. The MCOs will typically expect daily attendance by the patient in the program and may refuse to approve any more days if a patient has multiple absences. As a result of the hegemony, patient stays tend to be shorter than in the other cohorts.

Both levels of care with this cohort will emphasize group therapy as the primary treatment modality. Neither level will have individual therapy as it is not a billable service for this cohort, but the clinician will meet individually with a patient to conduct case management and treatment planning.

The distinction between the PHP and IOP levels in this cohort is that the PHP patient has higher acuity and is under the care of a psychiatrist.[1] The PHP session typically starts in the morning and meets longer on a given day than the IOP level, because the patient is viewed as needing additional monitoring and services.[2]

---

[1] Routine labs, including drug screens and pregnancy tests, may also be a part of the treatment as a precursor to the administration of medication.

[2] PHP sessions must be held during the morning when psychiatrists are at the hospital.

If they have not been started on medication in the inpatient level of care, the course of treatment for patients in the higher PHP level of care includes being started on a trial of medication by a psychiatrist. The patient is soon stepped down to the IOP level of care upon demonstration of medication tolerance or stability or when the MCO directs this.[3] This step-down is a formal discharge by the psychiatrist with an order to discharge and admit to the IOP level of care.

Patients in the IOP setting are viewed as having greater stability than PHP patients. The IOP patient is viewed as being unable to function normally and needs more intense therapy than can be provided in the typical outpatient setting.[4] Because a psychiatrist is not required for the IOP level of care, IOP sessions can also be held during the afternoon and at night.[5] When the patient has either demonstrated a reduction in acuity or the increased stability necessary to return to a normal routine, the patient is discharged from the IOP and normally referred to outpatient services.

This chapter covers working with the population of adults from age 18 to 65. It discusses the general treatment planning goals. It explores the provision of group therapy and psychoeducation. It examines family therapy, case management, discharge planning, and the unique problems found in this population.

TREATMENT PLANNING

Treatment planning with the adult PHP/IOP patient will closely resemble the discussion in Chapters 3 and 4. The clinician will likely prepare an initial treatment plan at admission and a concurrent treatment either at the designated interval or in conjunction with the next insurance or managed care review.

---

[3] The MCOs tend to move patients out of the PHP level quickly and approve far more IOP days.

[4] Some MCOs will pay only for IOP services. Some IOP patients present as needing medication checks, and the clinician may need to seek insurance authorization for a psychiatrist to see the patient.

[5] Medicare IOP patients are required to be under a psychiatrist's care and will have to attend during the morning.

Depending on the time constraints, the clinician will need to be brief but polite in conducting treatment planning sessions. The existing time constraint should be communicated to the patient. If a patient tries to convert the treatment planning session into an individual therapy session, the clinician should redirect the patient to discuss issues in the group therapy session.

As discussed in Chapter 3, the clinician may have to redirect the patient on what is reasonable in terms of goals. Many depressed and anxious patients overgeneralize and say that they want all of their problems gone. In these cases, the clinician has to prompt the patient as to what is realistic in the PHP/IOP, which includes the following:

- The patient will not resolve all of his or her problems but will get well enough to return to work.
- The patient will be evaluated for whether a medication is needed to address symptoms not resolvable by talk therapy.
- The patient will have an opportunity to talk about his or her problems and get support from the group.
- The patient will be introduced to various types of coping skills.

The clinician may then suggest some goals to the patient, such as:

- The patient will comply with medication as prescribed by the psychiatrist.
- The patient will talk in the group about personal stressors and issues.
- The patient will engage in a mood-improving activity outside of the group.

The clinician should solicit the patient for agreement on the treatment goals.

CASE MANAGEMENT

Along with treatment planning, the clinician will often have case management duties that include correspondence and completion of disability paperwork. Besides writing letters, the most typical paperwork will likely be Family and Medical Leave Act[6] forms. The next most common paperwork the clinician will complete is for short-term disability, which will vary in the extent of detail needed from simple form completion to performing mental status tests. Typically, the clinician will complete these documents for a psychiatrist to sign as many employers and disability insurance companies will only accept a physician's signature.[7]

At times, case management can include assisting the patient in locating financial assistance. The clinician may need to assist the patient in identifying charities or agencies that can assist in providing food, paying for prescription copays, and avoiding utility shutoff. Given all the clinician's duties, it is preferable to give a patient a list of potential resources so as to empower the patient to be responsible for addressing his or her problems.[8]

DISCHARGE PLANNING

Discharge planning with this population will follow along the lines discussed in Chapter 5. The clinician is typically the responsible party to make aftercare appointments for the patient as ordered by the psychiatrist or as suggested by the MCO. The reader is referred back to Chapter 5 for more detail.

---

[6] The Family and Medical Leave Act of 1993, or FMLA, is a U.S. law protecting adult patients or parents with children who require medical services. The Act does have parameters, such as the size of the employing organization and the length of employment prior to admission for treatment.

[7] If the patient was admitted to the IOP level from the community, the clinician may be able to sign the FMLA forms. If a psychiatrist's signature is required by the employer or disability insurance carrier, the clinician may need to get the insurance company or MCO to approve a medication check so that a psychiatrist can see the patient and sign the documents.

[8] How much a clinician decides to engage in financial assistance and social service work is a judgment call. It is helpful to identify a policy establishing the extent to which the clinician or treatment team will go in financial assistance work. Some patients present their problems as crises that prove to be the logical consequence of the patients' negligence. These patients may engage in staff splitting by claiming the primary clinician has not done anything for them regarding the problem.

GROUP THERAPY

Group therapy with the adult population will closely follow the clinician-facilitated process type described in Chapter 6. This particular cohort tends to do well with insight-oriented process therapy. Assuming that the PHP and IOP patients are served together, the process group can be very intense if not labile due to the acuity of the patients. If the PHP and IOP patients are served separately, the PHP group will be lower functioning and will require more clinician interaction.

As discussed in Chapter 6, group therapy can resemble individual therapy within the group session, because the patients are expected to talk about the problems that brought them into treatment. The patients, as group members, are directed to listen and to give each other empathetic feedback about problems and issues. Group therapy with this population has the potential to be an effective and efficient modality.

PSYCHOEDUCATION

Psychoeducation with this population closely follows the pattern discussed in Chapter 7. This population is best served with an organized rotation of psychoeducational subjects that relate to illness management, practical coping skills, and relationship issues. This population will likely appreciate handouts that the patients can review at a later date, which contain the salient points of the educational topics.

If the patient population is divided into PHP- and IOP-level groups, the PHP group will have a shorter rotation of psychoeducational sessions than the IOP group, and the presentations should be of a more basic nature, such as coping skills and illness management. If both levels are merged, only one psychoeducational rotation is required.

Regardless of whether the levels are merged, the PHP patients will typically have one more educational session in the afternoon before the patients leave for the day. This PHP education should be light, positive, practical, and not repeat the morning sessions.[9]

---

[9] This education should not be about dark subjects such as grief and loss.

FAMILY THERAPY

Family therapy is not common with the PHP/IOP adult cohort. The need for a family therapy session will be identified in the course of treatment planning, group therapy, or as mandated by an MCO reviewer.[10]

Family therapy is of limited value in the adult cohort, as there will be only one or two sessions. The session will only be able to address the most critical issues at hand. The stance of the clinician in this type of family session tends to be more that of an educator about symptoms, medication, and treatment than of an actual change agent. Relevant subjects for the family session include:

- Helping the family understand the patient's mental health issues
- Allowing family members who are stressed by the patient's mental health issues to talk about their feelings
- Developing a plan for how the family can support the patient's recovery
- Addressing specific issues of conflict or stress, such as the problems that existed at the time of the patient's admission

The family session attendees could be just the patient's spouse/significant other or other family members who are available and willing to participate.

An inherent problem with initial family sessions is that the participants can get overly emotional and the discussion never gets to the desired outcomes. Furthermore, one or more family members can attempt to triangulate the clinician into taking sides on an issue. A solution to this problem is to have structured family sessions.

Before the structured family session, the clinician and patient should briefly meet to discuss expectations. The discussion topics should include:

- Gaining a mutual understanding of the session's purpose and desired outcomes

---

[10] As discussed in Chapter 4, an MCO reviewer will indicate that a family session be conducted by the time of the next review. The MCO reviewer's rationale may be unknown, but if the family session is conducted, there is a risk that no further days will be approved and the patient will have to be discharged.

- Clarifying the patient's concerns about any specific family members and any particularly sensitive topics of significance
- Reviewing how the family session will be conducted

The presession meeting should be brief and will hopefully alleviate patient anxiety. A structured family session requires ground rules that the clinician reviews at the beginning of the session. These recommended ground rules include the following:

- This is a problem-solving session.
- I (the clinician) don't live in your house(s), and I do not see what goes on, so I cannot be the judge of who is right in "he said/she said" matters.[11]
- We will create a discussion list of subjects to which everyone will contribute.
- When we are done discussing the list items, we are done with the session.

After meeting all the session participants, the clinician should review the rules in the form of a preamble and then poll the participants for their concerns.

The wheel-spoke pattern of group interaction is helpful when structuring the family session. When there are more than two participants, the clinician should at least utilize it in the review of the list of concerns. When more than one participant has the same concerns, the first one who brought it up should be the one to start the discussion.

---

[11] Two family session participants can attempt to draw the clinician into a triangle of drama when they say the following:
"I'm right."
"No, I'm right."
"No, I'm right."
Then they look for the clinician to be the decision maker. If the clinician renders a judgment, the clinician becomes both a villain and a rescuer. Furthermore, one participant becomes a victim in the session, which could affect the productivity of the session. Application of this second rule helps to prevent this disruption. The clinician can say, "As I said at the beginning, I cannot be the judge of he said/ she said matters."

Depending on the spontaneity of the family members, the clinician can bring up the topics in order from the list and let the participants talk. If the participants are not being spontaneous, the clinician should utilize the wheel-spoke method. Although not every participant may have a comment, the clinician should monitor for who is not talking and prompt that participant for his or her view on the issue. When the discussion seems to be waning on a topic, the clinician should move to the next concern on the list.

When the list of topics has been completed, the clinician can poll the patient and family to see if they have any more topics. If they do not have any, the clinician should thank the family for coming in and supporting the patient and end the session.

It often is helpful for the clinician to follow up with the patient to get his or her feedback on the family session. The clinician and patient can then make a decision whether issues were satisfactorily addressed or another session is needed.

UNIQUE PROBLEMS

The unique problems of the adult PHP/IOP cohort are its wide age range, social diversity, and the presence of patients with personality disorders who are higher functioning. Because of these problems, the milieu can be intense and stressful.

The most prevalent of the three problems is that higher functioning personality-disordered patients may manifest entitlement, significant emotional lability, and sophistication in the instigation of drama. The patient with a personality disorder will often fire a clinician and/or demand to change groups because of feeling uncomfortable with the clinician. There is a further discussion on patients with personality disorders in Chapter 14.

The intensity of the drama can reach crisis levels depending on the point of contention and how far a patient pushes it. The drama will escalate if the staff and supervisor lack the emotional intelligence to identify and appreciate the drama for what it is, or if the supervisor does not support the staff in managing the drama. Possible consequences of escalated drama include increased patient absences and passive patient discharges, meaning patients do not return for treatment.

The personality-disordered patient in the adult cohort tests the cohesion of the treatment team and the supervisor's support for the clinician and staff. Dealing with the first personality-disordered patient as a team is an initiation into how things are done by other team members and by management. The clinician and team's learning curve may be in itself stressful as they learn each other's attitudes, limits, personalities, and knowledge base in responding to personality-disordered patients.

Diversity in the adult cohort is potentially a significant problem in that there can be patients from a wide variety of socioeconomic and educational backgrounds and developmental stages.[12] At any one time, the group can consist of factory workers, stay-at-home parents, and professionals. The group can also include both adults close to retirement age and patients in their 20s. The group could have high school dropouts and patients with PhDs. The clinician and staff will have the challenge of delivering services to all of the patients in a way that meets each patient's needs.

This problem is easier to negotiate because anxiety and depression cross all socioeconomic, educational, and ethnic lines. The patients in this program can talk about their symptoms and can relate to one another in terms of family and relationship stressors. The clinician may have to emphasize patient commonality in the midst of diversity and why patients are being treated when diversity becomes a point of conflict.

CONCLUSIONS

This chapter discussed practice with the PHP/IOP cohort of adults from age 18 to 64. It is the highest functioning cohort that tends to be the purest population for utilizing the different game strategies discussed in the earlier chapters. The work of the clinician with this population will be primary group therapy, psychoeducation, case management, and discharge planning.

Family therapy will be an occasional service in this cohort that the clinician will need to provide when the case calls for it or the MCO directs that a session be held. This chapter discussed a strategy for a structured

---

[12] The patients who tend to have a greater likelihood of intolerance are personality-disordered patients.

family session that aims to increase the likelihood that family members will stay on the task in addressing concerns and not get carried away by emotion. It is in both the patient's and the clinician's interests to ensure that this session is orderly, given that there will likely be only one family session.

The adult PHP/IOP milieu can be intense because of the higher level of acuity, but its unique challenges can make it seem more intense depending on the presence of acting-out behaviors by patients with personality disorders. This combination of acuity and acting out requires that the clinician and colleagues cooperate to manage the intensity.

Sometimes the clinician and his or her colleagues will have to make some kind of allowance or provision for diversity. However, regardless of the diversity, the patients who come into the PHP/IOP setting typically all have the same problems of mood and anxiety issues, which offers a common base to build on for meaningful clinical work.

Even with its intensity and challenges, the patients in the adult PHP/IOP cohort tend to respond well to treatment. It is a cohort in which the clinician will likely see much treatment success and in turn feel an increased sense of competence and intrinsic reward.

CHAPTER TEN

THE GERIATRIC/OLDER ADULT COHORT

The geriatric or older adult partial hospitalization program (PHP)/ intensive outpatient program (IOP) cohort serves patients aged 65 and older who are generally retired and not working.[1] These are not merely adults who are older; this is a different cohort. The older adult PHP/ IOP milieu may be the most socioeconomically diverse as it may have patients who are retired physicians and widowed blue-collar housewives with little education. Despite the diversity within itself, the older adult patient cohort does not particularly relate to the younger adult cohort.

The older adult patient may be a step-down from inpatient care, but could also be a direct admission from the community.[2] If the patient is a direct admission from the community, he or she will likely start a trial of medication as prescribed by a psychiatrist and will take part in group therapy.

Many patients in the older adult cohort may not be as accustomed to seeking mental health services as younger adults. Talking about feelings and problems may be foreign to these patients. Many of these patients are coerced by family members, caretakers, and physicians to get treatment, and they tend to be hesitant to participate at admission.

The older adult PHP/IOP setting tends to be most appropriate for patients with mood and anxiety issues who are physically and cognitively

---

[1] The distinction between older adults and adults is driven by managed care and utilization management.

[2] Older adults are often admitted to a geropsychiatric inpatient unit as opposed to a regular adult unit. Some hospitals have a continuum of services for older adults. Older adults may be at too low a level of functioning to be in a regular inpatient unit. They may also require fall precautions to which an older adult unit can cater.

capable of participating in group therapy and retaining information from day to day. The patient should be physically healthy or strong enough to come into the program and participate for its duration.[3]

Patients with dementia and psychosis can be served in the PHP/IOP if the patient's symptoms are mild. In this case, the patient does not have florid psychosis, and he or she is in the early stages of dementia and has the capability to participate meaningfully. The severity of dementia impairs a patient's ability to retain information and participate appropriately in treatment. A patient should be screened using an instrument such as the Mini–Mental State Examination to determine any impairment.

The older adult PHP/IOP milieu is quieter than others because the patients tend to have lower energy levels and tire easily. It does not have the intense drama and lability of the adult (ages 18–64) milieu and it cannot handle the disruptive, lower functioning patients with schizophrenia and severe personality disorders. If treatment is indicated and, if physically capable, such lower functioning older adult patients should be referred to a PHP/IOP for severely mentally ill patients.

In the United States, Medicare tends to be the driver of how the older adult PHP/IOP operates, as the majority of patients have Medicare Part B[4] or Medicare supplement insurance.[5] Medicare has rules[6] for PHP and IOP that include:

- A group size limit of 10 patients
- Both PHP and IOP patients must be under the care of a psychiatrist
- Only certain credentials can bill for services

---

[3] In the United States, the program must also be handicapped accessible in accordance with federal law and typical accreditation standards.

[4] As it pertains to Medicare in the United States, Medicare Part A is for inpatient hospital services. Medicare Part B is for outpatient services. As noted earlier, Medicare is also the name of the national health insurance in Canada.

[5] With Medicare, patients can stay as long as they meet the criteria for services. As a result, some patients may attend the PHP/IOP sessions for months.

[6] These rules can be found in local coverage determination documents on the website of the "fiscal intermediary" for a particular state. The fiscal intermediary is a federal government contractor who administers Medicare for a particular state or region.

- Only certain services can be billed
- A separate service/treatment note must be written for each hour of group therapy[7]

Given that both PHP and IOP patients are under the care of a psychiatrist, the distinction between the two levels tends to be how much time a patient spends in the program each week.[8]

The PHP level of care can be tiring and, given the Medicare copay, it can be expensive for the older adult patient. Given this consideration, many patients are stepped down quickly to the IOP because the psychiatrist is still supervising the patient's case. PHP tends to be especially reserved for those older adult cases of significantly higher acuity for which more observation is necessary.

Typically, the older adult patient is ready for discharge when it has been determined that the patient has maximized benefit from the program or is requesting to be discharged. The patient and his or her family members will hopefully have agreed that the patient's symptoms have improved and they have come to a consensus on a discharge plan.

This chapter discusses clinical work with the geriatric/older adult PHP/IOP cohort, aged 65 and older, and the application of the previously discussed games. It reviews the cohort's age-related issues, which include an interplay of medical problems and dementia. It covers the younger clinician's challenges in assuming the role of helper with this population. Applications of the games of treatment planning and group therapy are reviewed. It closes with a discussion of discharge planning.

THE PATIENT CHALLENGES

Patients in the older adult cohort have different life situations, concerns, and issues than the adult (age 18–64) cohort. These patients have been or are starting to transition into a new stage of life in which the identity they

---

[7] Commercial insurance will allow for one note to cover more than 1 hour of group therapy.

[8] The PHP patient will stay for all program hours 5 days per week, but there are two likely IOP formats. IOP patients can leave after 3 hours per day or stay for all program hours.

had for decades is lost with retirement. They may develop an increasing number of medical conditions that affect their mobility and functioning. The patients may be developing dementia and have increasing levels of frustration and grief due to the condition. It is a time when they may reflect on their vulnerability and grieve the loss of independence and control. Their adult children who did not turn out as hoped tend to be a source of guilt feelings and worry. This section elaborates on those concerns.

Older adults do not necessarily relate to younger adults who are struggling with work and family. They have different struggles that include deciding what they are going to do with themselves in retirement and developing a new identity as they have lost their primary identities. Part of their work in therapy may be grieving the loss of identity and finding new ways to be productive and have meaning in their lives.

Older adults decline in function and physical health and develop more and more medical conditions that are both stressors and causes of mental health symptoms.[9] They may be going to several specialists and taking a plethora of medications for a number of chronic conditions that have depression and anxiety as side effects. Some older adults may have had the onset of a new physical condition that has radically changed their lives, such as diabetes or cancer. Many older adults have more and more sources of chronic pain, which diminish their quality of life throughout the day. Sometimes, the different medical conditions complicate each other. As a result of all of the conditions and medications, much of their week may be spent in physicians' offices. It is not uncommon for patients to talk about their different medical problems in the group and socially with others.

Dementia is another medical condition connected with depression, anxiety, and psychosis that will be encountered in the older adult cohort. Dementia is a degenerative disease of the brain in which the patient experiences a decline in memory and executive functioning and some disorganized thought content.[10] The patient with dementia may also have both

---

[9] Urinary tract infections can precipitate psychotic episodes. Furthermore, some medications the patients take for general medical conditions may have depression as a side effect.

[10] There are numerous types of dementia. The two most common are the Lewy body and Alzheimer type. Dementia also can be caused by stroke, oxygen deprivation, anesthesia, and taking too much prescribed medication.

delusions and hallucinations. The older adult PHP/IOP cohort can serve patients with mild dementia or cognitive impairment.[11]

There often tends to be an interplay between dementia and anxiety. An older patient with dementia often evidences circumstantial thinking and difficulty developing insight regarding his or her problem. The patient may have problems practicing cognitive behavioral coping skills. He or she may develop both frustration and fear with the realization of lost capabilities, including remembering therapeutic concepts. The patient may talk about this condition in treatment.

In light of the medical conditions, many older adult patients in the PHP/IOP setting will discuss feelings of grief relating to their loss of independence and increased vulnerability. Some patients attempt to compensate for their health problems so as to maintain independence.[12] They may have hidden the facts about their true functioning level out of fear of losing their home and investments to pay for nursing home care. Many patients fight with their families over moving into assisted living or retirement housing because they want to stay in their own homes. When they have given into the reality that they must move out of the residence where they have spent their lives, the patients experience depression. They will often talk about this in the PHP/IOP setting.

Some patients present with strong feelings about other family issues, including adult children who did not turn out well. The adult children may be drug addicts and/or engaged in criminal activities. Patients will struggle with guilt and shame and dwell on where they may have gone wrong. If they do not feel guilty, some patients will express anger about how other family members are being codependent in enabling the dysfunctional family members.

ASSUMING THE ROLE OF HELPER WITH THE OLDER ADULT

Starting work with this population can be an awkward adjustment for the beginning or younger clinician who has had little contact with older adults other than grandparents and elders in churches or synagogues.

---

[11] This would be determined through a Mini–Mental State Examination.

[12] An example of this compensation occurs when patients taking diuretics to address edema and heart failure and who have a fear of falling will reduce their water consumption to reduce the number of bathroom trips and thus reduce their fall risks.

Typically, the younger clinician has tended to look up to older adults with respect. Some clinicians may have a mind-set that older adults know more than the clinician does about life. Symbolically, the clinician may be experiencing a rite of passage by assuming a helper role with the older adult patient.

Part of this rite of passage is a realization that some patients do not know more, nor do they possess more emotional maturity than the clinician. Living longer may not equal becoming wise or more emotionally mature. Older adults remain human beings who may not have learned everything there is to learn or they may not necessarily have reached emotional maturity. Nevertheless, the clinician may initially have to work through feelings of anxiety when interacting with older patients and becoming acclimated to a professional role in this setting.

On the other hand, many people have the unintentional habit of talking down in a parental tone to older adult patients with significant problems and smothering the older adult by trying to help with everything. This stance tends to arise from anxiety that the older adult is fragile. Many older adults respond to such condescension in a hostile, frustrated, or defensive fashion as their personal boundaries are crossed and their dignity is attacked; they are not children and do not want to be treated as such. The resulting defensiveness often gets wrongly translated into the patient exhibiting problems with anger.

The clinician should respect boundaries in general by treating older adult patients as adults with self-determination. In terms of transactional analysis, the clinician's communication should be that of an adult to another adult. If a patient appears to be struggling when ambulating, the clinician should ask whether the patient needs help before touching the patient. Furthermore, the clinician should ask the patient how much help the patient wants. This respect of boundaries is therapeutic for the older adult patient and can open the door for more productive therapy.

Another challenging growth experience in beginning to work with this population is that some older adults may display and express awkwardness in talking to a clinician young enough to be a grandchild. In addition to communicating on the adult level, the clinician should validate the patient's feelings, express empathy for the situation, and proceed with treatment planning or the group session. Although there may be hesitation on the part of the patient to self-disclose at the initial contact (whether it be group therapy or treatment planning), it is important for the clinician to proceed in an adult and objective manner with the group session and treatment planning session. Some patients may never get over the awkwardness, but as long as the essential clinical tasks are completed and a relevant treatment plan is created, the clinician is successful.

TREATMENT PLANNING

Treatment planning with this cohort tends to have more family involvement than the other adult cohorts. The patient is often accompanied at admission by a spouse and/or or adult child. These family members provide input that includes both their concerns and details about the patient's problems. How concurrent treatment planning is conducted is based on the variables of patient conditions and issues, family assertiveness,[13] program policy, and psychiatrist preference. Otherwise, the treatment planning processes tend to deviate little from the descriptions provided in Chapters 3 and 4.

DISCHARGE PLANNING

Discharge planning for the older adult cohort tends to be simpler than it is for the younger cohorts, but it is not necessarily easier. Older adults rarely follow up with an individual therapist, but may follow up with the psychiatrist.[14] The majority of older adult patients tend to follow up with their primary care physician for medication management. Many patients will have mental health care and medication management through home health agencies. Much of the clinician's discharge planning will be helping older adult patients identify senior day programs where they are willing to go to socialize and avoid isolation.

---

[13] Some patients have active and concerned family members who act as caretakers, powers of attorney, and maybe even guardians. Consultation with these family members is crucial to treatment and discharge planning.

[14] Psychiatrists may have different practice policies in their offices and may take only patients with Medicare supplement insurance.

GROUP THERAPY AND PSYCHOEDUCATION

Group therapy with the older adult in the PHP/IOP setting tends to be a process group and not a memory group.[15] The process group tends to be an effective arena for patients to self-disclose anxieties, grief issues, and other stressors. Patients also gain from identifying with others who have similar problems. Moreover, it is a favorable format for the clinician to facilitate problem-solving discussions.

This cohort often requires the clinician to be an active group leader, given the various aforementioned reasons. This includes engaging in an extended wheel-spoke pattern to catalyze a group process in which the clinician attempts to get patients to give more detail about why they were admitted and to disclose their primary stressors. The clinician's work may include repeated efforts to normalize feelings such as anxiety and anger. He or she may also have to go into detail empathizing with the patients on otherwise simple issues that become big issues for older adults, such as getting to the bathroom without falling. Otherwise, much of the material in Chapter 6 on process group therapy is applicable to this cohort.[16]

On the other hand, psychoeducation with this cohort is different from the adult (18–64 years) cohort. Many, but not all, of the same subjects are applicable to the older adult cohort.[17] Furthermore, depending on the level of dementia among patients, the material and its presentation may need to be concrete, experiential, and expressive. This cohort may benefit more from a relaxation exercise than a lecture on relaxation techniques.

---

[15] The memory group is essentially a mood-improving exercise in which patients are encouraged to think back to good times, which results in positive emotions.

[16] If there is more than one group and more than one clinician in a program, clinicians may choose to switch groups for variety for both the patients and the clinicians at the end of a therapy hour. If this is the case, clinicians will need to brief each other during the break as to the significant clinical issues discussed in the group.

[17] Cognitive behavioral therapy and self-care are examples of appropriate topics, but topics about coping at work are not applicable for older adults.

FAMILY THERAPY

Family therapy is relatively common in the older adult cohort. Family sessions are often held concerning the decision to move the patient out of his or her house and into assisted or senior living. Other family sessions are held to educate family members about mental health issues and treatment. It is also a platform for helping family members understand what kind of role they can play in the patient's recovery. The strategy for conducting family sessions discussed in Chapter 9 works well with this cohort.

CONCLUSIONS

This chapter discussed clinical work in the older adult PHP/IOP cohort. Patients in this cohort experience an interplay among medical problems, dementia, and mental health problems, which are regular subjects in therapy. A younger clinician beginning to work with this cohort may struggle to adjust to the professional role, given that the patients may be the age of a grandparent. Treatment- and discharge-planning processes with this cohort are similar to the other adult cohorts. The tendency for family involvement in both treatment planning and treatment itself will be higher than with the other adult cohorts because crucial and unpleasant decisions have to be made about the patient's living arrangements. The PHP/IOP setting has the potential to serve a pivotal role in the lives of older adults.

   The older adult population is a distinct cohort with different developmental needs and different stressors. As they age and experience diminished functioning, matters that had been simple and problem free in their earlier years cause difficulties for these patients. Although they can develop clinical depression and anxiety problems, older adults experience stress over diminished mobility, cognitive functioning, and increased medical problems. They suffer grief and loss over many issues that vary from the death of a spouse and loss of a career to retirement and to the ability to get in and out of a bathtub by themselves. Although it may be necessary for a patient to give up living independently and move into assisted living or a nursing home, this presents another significant loss. The PHP/IOP setting has great potential to help older adult patients cope with these difficult decisions and issues.

The older adult PHP/IOP also has the potential to be a very rewarding but challenging setting in which to work. It is often meaningful to assist patients and families in navigating crucial and painful decisions. This is a setting where a clinician can grow personally and professionally by developing different skills while helping struggling people who are in a later stage of life, which the clinician will likely enter. It is often an opportunity for a clinician to appreciate personal mortality and its result ing implications for personal values and priorities.

CHAPTER ELEVEN

THE CHRONICALLY MENTALLY ILL

*T*he chronically mentally ill, also referred to as those with severe and persistent mental illness, was essentially the original cohort for whom partial hospitalization was created. Partial hospitalization is an economical option that allows patients to continue treatment while having a higher quality of life outside the inpatient unit.

Patients appropriate for the partial hospitalization program (PHP)/ intensive outpatient program (IOP) levels of care in this cohort should be of a high-enough functioning level to participate. A patient should be cognitively intact and attend to his hygiene and general activities of daily living. A patient appropriate for the PHP/IOP should have the self-control to sit in a therapy group and to participate meaningfully. Furthermore, the patient should show some motivation to be treatment compliant.

The patient with a chronic mental illness served in a PHP/IOP setting is typically on disability for it. Patients with chronic mental illness may have diagnoses of schizophrenia, schizoaffective disorder, bipolar disorder, and major depressive disorder, among others. Patients who have severe personality-disorder traits may also be served in this program. Some of the patients meet the criteria for the diagnoses of both a mental illness and a personality disorder. The expectations for this type of patient are lower because of the symptomology and the patient's lower distress tolerance, which makes it difficult for the patient to engage in intense psychotherapy.

A younger patient experiencing an initial schizophrenic break may also be served in this program. The patient and family may be coming to terms with the reality of his or her life-changing condition, which includes a grief-and-loss process. This patient's grief and loss often includes a period of denial involving multiple hospitalizations until the patient accepts the illness and the need for medication to manage the symptoms.

The overall program emphasis is to stabilize the patient sufficiently so he or she will return to baseline level. In this cohort, a patient may continue to have significant symptomology at the time of discharge, which may include hallucinations and paranoia, but the treatment team strives to manage the patient's symptoms until the patient is back at baseline. The patient is typically referred back to the local public mental health clinic or agency for the continued management of symptoms.

The length of patient stay in the PHP/IOP is based on the payer source. The majority of patients in this cohort depend on public insurance. In the United States, the patient who has only Medicare B could stay until the psychiatrist and treatment team have determined that the patient is at baseline or has maximized possible benefits of treatment and no longer meets the criteria for treatment. The drawback with Medicare is that the patient has a copay and may incur unsupportable debt unless the hospital has a financial assistance policy.[1] The patient with commercial insurance will likely have a short stay. With the rise of managed Medicaid,[2] the patient with this coverage will not be liable for any copays but will also tend to have a shorter stay due to utilization review.

As with the older adult cohort, the patient with Medicare will have a psychiatrist in the IOP setting.[3] Unless the patient has a number of pre-approved days at the PHP level, it is likely that step-down to the IOP level will be rapid.

This chapter discusses working with the chronically mentally ill cohort in the PHP/IOP setting. It discusses the treatment challenges and applications of the games used with this cohort.

---

[1] Patients with severe mental illness typically receive Social Security, Medicaid, and Medicare. There are limits as to how much additional income they can earn without penalty. Therefore, they tend to be unable to afford the standard out-of-pocket copay required with Medicare. Medicaid tends to pay 100% of the cost of PHP/IOP services.

[2] Medicare is an entitlement based on disability or age. Medicaid is a means-tested entitlement based on the income of the patient. The presence of Medicaid and Medicare patients depends on the agency or hospital's contracts to take such patients.

[3] The IOP patient with Medicaid may have a psychiatrist based on the provider contract with the state or managed care organization (MCO).

POPULATION-RELATED CHALLENGES
AND EXPECTATIONS

There are a number of challenges in working with chronically mentally ill patients in the PHP/IOP. Group therapy can be difficult with this population, and it tends to be of limited value, given the nature of the chronic conditions. Like group therapy, treatment planning can be difficult depending on the poverty of thought, concrete thinking, or paranoia of a patient. Patients may be noncompliant with medication due to side effects or because they start believing they simply do not need it. Another challenge occurs when a patient uses alcohol and drugs that interfere with medications and cause additional psychiatric symptoms. Last, but not the least, finding structure and meaning can be a struggle for this population as the average patient may have few personal resources and an overabundance of free time. The clinician should take these challenges into account when approaching and interacting with the patients.

It is imperative that the clinician demonstrate calmness, patience, and a low-key approach with this cohort. It should be assumed that the patients are not intentionally slow to answer, but that their illnesses are creating some kind of cognitive impairment or hesitation. An anxious clinician unable to tolerate patient silence or hesitation may unintentionally monopolize the conversation, which turns process therapy groups and treatment planning sessions into lectures.

In light of low patient functioning, the milieu of this particular PHP/IOP appears to be a background element versus an element that has a meaningful impact on the patient's recovery. The milieu becomes a factor when there are bizarrely disruptive[4] or antisocial patients who intimidate or scare other patients who are already paranoid. Otherwise, the majority of the patients in this cohort tend to have an acceptance, if not tolerance, for mildly bizarre and psychotic behavior. In general, management of the milieu in this PHP/IOP cohort is a matter of maintaining order and peace while accepting benign psychotic behavior.

---

[4] An example of bizarrely disruptive behavior is the pseudoseizure, which is a form of panic attack.

TREATMENT PLANNING GOALS

The overall goal for the patient in this PHP/IOP cohort is to demonstrate stability. Stability includes patient compliance with medication and reports of using one or more alternative coping skills. An important aspect of stability is that the patient is observed to evidence some improvement or amelioration in affective presentation. If the patient does not have reduced symptoms and improvement in affect, stability would include no regression.

At face value, the starting point for treatment planning is the patient's functioning level. If the patient is unable to identify any particular goals, the clinician may need to reverse the line of questioning and seek to identify what the patient does not want to happen again and then what it will take to prevent that from happening. If the patient still cannot identify any particular areas, it may be helpful to ask what the patient understands to be the reason for referral to the PHP/IOP. If the patient is still unable to identify treatment goals, the clinician should suggest two or three basic goals that fit the program design.

Typical patient goals will include the following:

- The patient will be compliant with the medication as prescribed by the psychiatrist.
- The patient will attend the program and participate in group therapy sessions.
- The patient will identify two symptom triggers.
- The patient will perform daily hygiene and activities of daily living.
- The patient will identify and engage in some legal mood-improving activity.
- The patient will abstain from the use of alcohol and drugs.

Often, the hospital or organization has a set of predetermined goals that are already supplied for use in this program.

GROUP THERAPY

Group therapy with the chronically mentally ill can be an experience of extremes. Sometimes the group as a whole can be withdrawn due to vegetative mood symptoms, anxiety, or paranoia. On the other hand, the group may be noisy and euphoric when a number of patients are simultaneously manic and impulsive. It can be high-strung when there are a number of paranoid patients who are verbal. The group may be full of drama when there is a higher prevalence of personality-disordered patients who are intolerant of each other. The successful clinician will develop and demonstrate a set of skills for each scenario.

The scenario of the withdrawn group seems to drain the most energy from the clinician. Besides vegetative or severe mood symptoms, the patients may not have much to discuss. In light of this difficulty, the beginning clinician may experience serious self-doubt about his or her capability of performing group therapy in this situation.

A helpful approach in the withdrawn group is to use a repeated wheel-spoke approach, by going around the room and seeking to involve each of the group members in whatever topic is being discussed. When a patient steps up and engages in spontaneous discussion or disclosure, the clinician can seek general group feedback or repeat the wheel-spoke strategy.

The opposite experience occurs when the group is full of patients with mania. The clinician's challenge will not be getting patients to talk but maintaining group order and redirecting patients from talking about inappropriate subjects.

The group that is full of verbal, delusional patients presents a different challenge for the clinician. The clinician may attempt to engage a paranoid patient in problem solving and identification of coping skills only to realize that the patient is delusional because he or she does not seem to connect or that he or she sounds like a broken record. On the other hand, some patients with obvious religious delusions may need to be allowed to talk until the point that either they are being inappropriate or they are monopolizing the group. It is crucial for the clinician to maintain calm composure and roll with the delusions in a group and keep the group discussion going.[5]

---

[5] Opinions vary as to whether or not delusional patients should be confronted about delusions. In the interest of milieu management and respect for the patient, it is best that patients at least not be confronted about delusions in the group setting. If a patient becomes labile or agitated in discussion about delusional material, he or she should be excused from the group to calm down.

When a group in this cohort tends to have a predominance of personality-disordered patients, the likelihood exists that the clinician will walk into the middle of the drama and patient–staff splitting. The patient claiming to be victimized or disrespected may identify another patient as a rude and offending villain or perpetrator. One or more patients may target an identified pariah and collectively storm out even if the clinician tries to process the problem and seek its resolution in the group.

In the end, group therapy in this cohort can at times seem to be more of an opportunity to monitor patients for acuity than it is for improving patient insight and coping skills. When the group is a withdrawn group, the clinician should focus on documenting patient symptomology and the patients' lack of participation.

PSYCHOEDUCATION

Meaningful psychoeducation with this cohort can be a challenge because of redundancy. Some patients have heard the same topics repeatedly, because either they have been in the program repeatedly or they have been enrolled for an extended time of months or years. It is difficult to have an education rotation of any length for this cohort without redundancy. However, many of the patients will not complain when they have heard the same topic repeatedly. The clinicians will likely feel the awkwardness over the redundancy more than the patients.

Some of the awkwardness may be out of a confined view of what is appropriate education for this cohort, such as medication compliance and basic coping skills. With the confined view, there is an inherent danger of patronizing patients, which can precipitate noncompliance. Even though they have chronic conditions that make them low functioning, the patients live in the real world and have real problems.

Many of the same educational topics used in the regular adult cohort are appropriate for the chronically mentally ill but may need to be revised into more basic terms. The educational topics not applicable may have to do with work environments, but patients in this cohort may still benefit from learning about relationships, family systems, goal setting, and time management in addition to self-care and illness management.

FAMILY THERAPY

Family involvement in this cohort tends to be sparse except in cases of younger patients having their first psychotic break. Most of the time, the patient tends to be detached from family members due to family conflict or weariness of the family members from years of dealing with the patient's needs and problems.

Whatever family sessions occur in this cohort tend to be pointed. The reason for the session tends to be clear from the outset and hopefully a plan for supporting the patient's treatment is an outcome. A typical reason for a family session is to help the younger patient and family understand the illness and the typical course of treatment. The older chronic patient rarely presents with family issues and family members who are available and willing to come in for sessions.

DISCHARGE PLANNING

The discharge plan for the typical patient in this cohort is practically predetermined as follow-up at the local public mental health agency. In larger metropolitan areas, there may be a private practice or medical school training clinic that takes this population. However, the public mental health agency will more likely be the patient's only option.

The two likely problems with discharge planning in this cohort are the patient's noncompliance with follow-up and the patient's resistance to returning to a therapist with whom he or she has had conflict. Many patients may have irresolvable conflict with their outpatient therapists and do not want to go back to them. On the other hand, many patients fail to follow up with outpatient treatment and are eventually rehospitalized. The reality is that the clinician cannot coerce a patient to follow through with aftercare.

The clinician can explore a patient's resistance to follow up with the public mental health provider and determine whether the patient can be referred to a different therapist and/or psychiatrist within that agency. Depending on how complex and open the public mental health provider is, the clinician may be able to reach the designated therapist or case manager and advocate for the patient.[6]

The clinician may have to contact the available family to play a part in a patient's follow-up. Sometimes the family can be a strong influence on the patient to keep appointments and perhaps go with the patient back to the agency for readmission. The clinician is limited in terms of options and will have to follow protocol by making aftercare appointments for the patient. The clinician should discuss this limit with the patient and possibly the patient's family members. It will be up to the patient and possibly the family to persuade the patient to follow up and keep outpatient appointments.

CONCLUSIONS

This chapter discussed working with the chronically mentally ill cohort in the PHP/IOP setting. It is a low-functioning cohort that requires a clinician to have a patient and low-key approach. Because of functioning issues, group therapy in this cohort at times may serve more of a monitoring function than a treatment modality. Acceptance of redundancy in psychoeducation may be required, given how long patients may stay in the program. Treatment planning may require more clinician prompting than is ideal, given the patient's low functioning or passiveness. Discharge planning will likely be limited, because in any given locality, there are few outpatient providers who serve the chronically mentally ill. Although there is a desire to empower the patient's self-determination in as many areas as possible, the clinician may have to elucidate the treatment and discharge options for the patient.

---

[6] There are several problems in advocating in these situations. First, the patient may be a poor historian and not remember the outpatient therapist's name. The patient may be discharged from the agency due to noncompliance and the patient would have to be readmitted, so the patient technically will not have an official case manager, therapist, and psychiatrist (and so there is no one to talk to). Third, the therapist or case manager may not return phone calls. Fourth, the clinician may walk into a drama between the patient and the outpatient therapist in which both claim to be victims or both claim the other is a villain (which means problem solving is unlikely).

This particular cohort has the greatest stigma of all the cohorts. Many people are afraid of the chronically mentally ill. The fear has a modicum of validity because of the various publicized violent crimes committed by individuals with severe and persistent mental illness. However, these are patients who deserve respect and dignity. The clinician is in a position to give a patient with a chronic mental illness the therapeutic dignity and respect that others will not.

CHAPTER TWELVE

CHILDREN AND ADOLESCENTS

The child–adolescent partial hospitalization program (PHP)/intensive outpatient program (IOP) is for children and adolescents of school age who meet the symptom criteria. During the school year, these patients are unable to function in the regular school setting due to psychiatric issues. The patient in this cohort is sufficiently safe and stable enough to be at home at night and not in need of 24-hour inpatient treatment. The patient must also have at least average intelligence so as to be capable of understanding treatment. This is typically the only PHP/IOP cohort that is kept in a locked unit where the staff can refuse to let a patient leave.[1]

Children and adolescents tend to be lumped together in one general cohort for the purposes of Medicaid billing. However, they comprise three different subcohorts with different cognitive levels and abilities. The basic cohorts are child (5–9 years), preteen (10–12 years), and adolescent (13–18 years).[2]

The lines between the different cohorts can be blurry. Some preteen patients are immature for their age and may best be served in the child cohort. Some 13-year-old patients may be better off in the preteen cohort. Depending on waiting lists and overall group immaturity, a 12-year-old could be served in the adolescent group.[3] The cohort boundaries depend on the current census and individual patient characteristics.

A variety of psychiatric problems can be treated in the child and adolescent PHP/IOP. The problems include impulsivity and behavior disorders, mood issues, anxiety issues,[4] and psychotic disorders. One

---

[1] Adults could be kept only if there is a doctor-ordered hold or a court order.

[2] These are suggested divisions.

[3] In this case, the adolescent population would probably have no patient over the age of 15.

[4] Anxiety issues can include school refusal and trauma/posttraumatic stress disorder (PTSD).

important variant in this cohort is school refusal, which presents as part behavior disorder and part anxiety disorder and in which truancy officials and child protection officials are involved.[5] A patient with eating disorders could be treated in the PHP/IOP if the patient has other psychiatric issues. The patient must be able to demonstrate capability and motivation in the program to attend and participate in all activities and sessions.

The child and adolescent PHP is distinct from the IOP in that the patient is under the care of a psychiatrist and the program lasts all day with more services. The services include school, group therapy, individual therapy, and family therapy.[6] Typically, the PHP is based in a hospital that collaborates with a public school district to hold a specific number of classroom hours each day.

The PHP can also be intense and chaotic based on the number of patients there who have behavior disorders and personality issues. Many of these patients have aggressive and disruptive anger problems that require the use of a quiet or secluded room. Staff may have to use physical restraints when patients are aggressive toward themselves and others. Given that it is a milieu, these aggressive patients often irritate and instigate each other and detract from treatment focus.

The child and adolescent IOP consists of either a half-day service where the patient comes into a PHP for half of the day or it is an afternoon/evening program that offers only group therapy and case management. The patient is considered to be of a lower acuity level, is not aggressive, and is more motivated to be in treatment than a PHP patient. The IOP does not require a psychiatrist, and it can be held as an after-school program in any appropriate site.

This chapter discusses the distinct challenges presented by this population. It discusses the differences among children, preteens, and adolescents and the implications for treatment planning and treatment goals for these groups. It discusses the inclusion of family and individual

---

[5] Some patients with school refusal evidence an anxiety disorder, whereas some of these patients are beyond the control of the parents. There is also a variant of the anxiety disorder/school refusal scenario in which a patient is enmeshed with a parent who has a personality disorder and both feed into each other's anxiety; both are anxious about the child going to school.

[6] Depending on the payer source, family therapy has a subtype called collateral therapy, which is only for the parents; the patient is not in the room.

therapy, the inclusion of the school as part of the milieu, and some unique problems that may need to be addressed.

THE DIFFERENCES AMONG CHILDREN, PRETEENS, AND ADOLESCENTS

As already noted, there are obvious age-related differences among the different child, preteen, and adolescent cohorts. They have different levels of cognitive development and different needs.

The patient in the child cohort is cognitively concrete, and the clinician interventions may be as much family based as they are individual. Although there may be some depression and suicidality present, impulsivity and aggression tend to be more common problems.[7] A typical child gains little insight from talk therapy and will benefit from individual play therapy or art therapy. The successful group therapy approach is group play for socialization and art therapy for expression. Family therapy is important for addressing behavioral issues in the home and for monitoring progress. This population may also benefit from behavior modification such as a token economy. The role of the psychiatrist coupled with medication management is more significant in the treatment of the child cohort than are the psychotherapies.

With some exceptions, the preteen cohort is slightly more abstract in its thought process and more verbal and, therefore, capable of some insight-based therapy whether it be in the group or in individual sessions. This cohort tends to have patients with mood, anxiety, impulsivity, and behavior disorders. The preteen cohort tends to be chaotic, given the immaturity and anxiety of middle school–aged patients when in a group of their peers. Because of this immaturity, these patients tend to be very competitive and frequently tease each other to the point of bullying or being abusive. It is in this cohort that attention-deficit issues stand out as disruptive in the group setting, given that there is a greater expectation of patients to sit still and take part in a cognitive activity.

Of the three groups, the adolescent cohort tends to have the most noticeable and dramatic variation in terms of cognitive ability, symptomology,

---

[7] This cohort may also have elimination disorders, such as encopresis, from time to time.

and maturity. This cohort contains patients with psychotic disorders, mood disorders, anxiety disorders, eating disorders, and behavior disorders. Some of the patients evidence substance use. The patients also manifest maximum contrast in emotional maturity and cognitive capacity, which has implications for the focus of therapy groups. With all these variations in patient presentation, the staff has the constant challenge of monitoring the milieu and continuously adjusting approaches and arrangements of groups so as to maximize its therapeutic value and reduce disruption.

THE CHALLENGES OF BEHAVIOR
DISORDERS IN THE PHP/IOP SETTING

No matter what the cohort, behavior-disordered patients tend to be an inordinate problem in a milieu. They openly challenge and mock staff, therapists, and other patients in group settings. This type of patient also tends to engage in bullying and attempted bullying of weaker patients and staff through direct and passive-aggressive behaviors.[8] These patients tend to be defiant, verbally aggressive, and threatening to staff and other patients. Their behavior can escalate to hitting, pushing, or throwing objects at staff and other patients. A program milieu with several behavior-disordered patients may provide the opportunity for these particular patients to form negative cliques that cooperate to disrupt and bully other patients to defocus from treatment. With all these complications, staff members are challenged to treat these patients and minimize their disruption of the milieu.

The behavior-disordered patient tends to have lower cognitive functioning with little motivation to change. In a psychoanalytical sense, this patient has poor ego functioning, including poor insight, poor distress tolerance, strong denial tendency,[9] and poor problem-solving skills.

---

[8] When bullying, the patient may engage in critical and intimidating behavior that crosses personal boundaries. The bullying tends to emanate from anger, anxiety, or boredom. The staff member who has the emotional intelligence to appreciate the bullying behavior can respond in a parental or adult way that controls the dynamics.

[9] With the denial tendency, the behavior-disordered patient takes little to no responsibility for behavior and readily blames others when confronted.

The behavior-disordered patient with attention deficit issues tends to be noncompliant with medication because of intolerance of the side effects.[10] The patient may also have a self-concept of being a criminal or aggressive person.

The behavior-disordered patient's behavior issues are complicated in cases of substance use. If the patient is beyond parental control, there is the continued likelihood that he or she will continue to use drugs throughout treatment. The patient's drug use impairs judgment and engenders continued mood disturbance, regardless of any medications that are prescribed.

There is further complication when the behavior-disordered patients come from dysfunctional family systems where the behavior has a role in the family's equilibrium. The patient may have one or more parent with mental illness, personality issues, or substance abuse, which translates as the parent having an impairment or insidious contradictory agenda that sabotages treatment.[11] The family may also concretely state that the patient's admission is for school attendance and not treatment.[12] The parental figures or caretakers may also be in the midst of their own crises or unfavorable situations that detract their attention from treatment. As a result of the dysfunction, the parents and family members have poor compliance and attendance and make frequent excuses for missing family sessions.

The bottom line with behavior-disordered patients and their families is that treatment will have to be looked at in terms of maximized benefit. Inherently, many of the families of behavior-disordered patients seek to use the PHP/IOP as a simple solution to a complex or complicated problem that is often beyond the scope of the program. Given this

---

[10] Attention deficit hyperactivity disorder (ADHD) is often an underlying symptom of behavior disorders. It does seem to require ego development on the part of the child or adolescent to tolerate the medication side effects and see the value of the medication.

[11] Sometimes the parent's insidious agenda may just be surreptitious, but there may actually be parents who have a malevolent intention.

[12] This problem may be foreshadowed in initial treatment planning when the patient and family state that school is the primary problem and that the goal is for the patient to attend school.

complex situation, the therapist and staff can find themselves working harder than the patient and family to make the solution fit the problem.

INDIVIDUAL THERAPY

The child and adolescent cohort is the only PHP/IOP cohort for which both family and individual therapy are program expectations. The other cohorts have optional family therapy but not individual therapy.

Individual therapy has the advantage of addressing sensitive patient issues that are too personal to be addressed in group sessions. It is also a therapeutic opportunity for the patient to disclose concerns. Depending on the level of rapport, the clinician can confront a patient about behavior issues or use motivational interviewing to stimulate a patient to talk about motivation for changing. Because of the short time frame available, individual therapy in the PHP/IOP tends to be brief and problem solving in nature.

The general challenge is that children and adolescents are not good candidates in general for individual therapy, given their cognitive and motivational levels. In general, a child between the ages of 5 and 9 may be able to tell that there is a problem in general and concrete terms, but the child will offer simple answers and is likely to be incapable of elaboration and insight. Preteen patients are a little more capable of talking about problems but tend to be guarded about issues. Adolescents tend to show more capability to engage in individual therapy, but this varies from case to case depending on the patient's individual functioning. It is generally a valid conclusion that a child or adolescent patient is not necessarily a willing individual therapy participant.

A more specific challenge of individual therapy occurs with behavior-disordered and some personality-disordered patients. This type of patient often does not have the motivation to change. These patients tend to be guarded and refuse to talk openly in sessions. If the clinician in turn is directive, asking specific questions, the patient will respond with minimal answers. Furthermore, the patient may be avoidant of individual sessions and instead confront a clinician in front of a crowd about issues and questions. Because many clinicians have job expectations to meet with patients in individual sessions on a weekly basis for a certain time length, the clinician will likely focus on having the patient talk about problems in the here and now and use play therapy as a softening tool to lessen the intensity of such sessions.

FAMILY THERAPY

As a usual expectation of the PHP/IOP, family therapy should offer the opportunity to assess whether the patient is safe and demonstrating improvement out in the community. The clinician ascertains from the parent or guardian the patient's progress and lingering issues and expresses what he or she considers to be the patient's remaining goals. The family sessions provide an opportunity to address the relevant patient problems occurring outside of the program. The clinician will hopefully help the parent identify options for dealing with problem situations.

The family session in the PHP/IOP may be the first significant conversation adolescents and their parents/guardians have after admission or even after the step-down from inpatient care to discuss the hospitalization and residual issues. The typical categories of family topics deal with patient behavior. If there is no behavioral issue, then the patient's mood, anxiety, and self-esteem are often a concern. The patient often wants to know what it will take to get lost privileges restored. The family session can be a vital component in treatment as the clinician guides the interaction and negotiation between the patient and guardian and/or family to find possible solutions to the identified problems.

Despite its possible benefits, family therapy in the PHP/IOP can be a challenge because many families are avoidant and noncompliant with it.[13] Some families are noncompliant out of the fear of family secrets being disclosed. Some of the noncompliance is indicative of the parent's or guardian's own disorganization and low functioning because some parents tend to be in constant chaos. One complicated reason for the noncompliance is that parents and other key family members are mentally ill or dysfunctional and have no interest in changing, and thus they do not make attendance a priority.

Parents and families display their avoidance in a number of passive-aggressive ways. On the days when family sessions are scheduled, the patient may not attend the program and the family will not answer phone calls. Another avoidant technique used is when the patient comes to the program

---

[13] When the patient is in foster care, there is the recurring scenario that foster parents have no interest in attending family sessions and have the backing of the legal guardian not to come. In such situations, the PHP is looked at only as a stabilization stage of treatment.

and relays the message that the parent cannot come for the session.[14] Some parents may at least call and leave a voice mail message that they cannot come but do not ask for rescheduling. A typical part of this avoidance is that the parents do not return the clinician's phone calls to reschedule a session.[15]

Family avoidance of therapy sessions is frustrating for a clinician trying to maintain productivity and clinical standards. Although the family sessions are an expectation, the clinician tends to have little leverage in persuading parents and family to show up for sessions. The clinician can tell the families that there is a risk of discharge if they do not comply, but this amounts to an empty threat when the decision rests with a detached psychiatrist. [16]

In addition to the avoidance, the emotionality of families interferes with the productivity of family sessions. The patient and family members are often defensive, tense, and apprehensive prior to the family session. The patient and family may have mutual anger that manifests in distractibility and tangential discussion of various hurts and peccadilloes instead of the actual issues of focus. If the family session is too stressful, it may lead to one or more participants leaving the room and refusing to return, as well as avoidance of coming to another session.

Related to emotionality is the problem-centered family that frames issues in vague and nebulous terms. The problem-centered family may

---

[14] A recurring pattern occurs in which, after the patient gives the message, his or her mother does not answer the phone for several days and does not return phone calls. When some mothers are eventually reached, they say, "I told them I was not going to be able to come to family sessions." This tends to be a form of parent–staff splitting and instigation of drama.

[15] Many families using Medicaid or public insurance may not have the money to pay for gasoline or public transit to come to family sessions.

[16] Even with the lack of family compliance, a psychiatrist may have a personal agenda or basic philosophy to try and work with a patient even if the family does not come. In terms of being principled and ethical, the standard for discharge should be whether the patient is benefitting from treatment without the family's participation. If a family complains about the patient's behavior at home and avoids family sessions, the central problem is not being addressed and the patient should be discharged. If the family is avoiding sessions and the patient is unmotivated and noncompliant with medication, the patient should be discharged. On the other hand, if the patient is benefitting from treatment despite the family's noncompliance, it seems ethical that the patient stay in treatment.

be chaotically enmeshed and conceptualize issues in emotional terms and drama. This family makes the patient a scapegoat for the sins of the family. The emotionally framed problem is not one that has a solution, such as "You have attitude." The clinician often has to clarify with the parent or family member bringing up the emotionally framed problem what "attitude" even means and what the specific behavioral problem to be resolved is.

A fourth challenge in family therapy is the dysfunctional parent who actually shows up to the family session but is not interested in exploring change. The parent may be treatment savvy and discount any clinician suggestion as having already been tried unsuccessfully. The parent may have no insight nor take responsibility for family issues contributing to the patient's problems. Such a parent may be inconsistent, have poor boundaries, use illicit substances, or have anger management problems, and may blame all personal problems on the child or adolescent. This type of family session makes for a frustrating, if not unproductive, hour.

These challenges to family therapy in the PHP/IOP setting are indicators that not all patients and families will benefit from the therapy. It is of no use if families do not attend. If the family puts up resistance in the forms of drama and nebulous problem definition, the family's goals will not get addressed.[17] If a treatment-savvy, dysfunctional parent spends most of the session telling the clinician why an option will not work, the parent is not truly interested in change. In the end, the best that clinicians can do in these limited situations is to document that family therapy was attempted.

A suggested game arising out of the challenges is a structured family session similar to the format discussed in Chapter 10. The modification of this format is an emphasis that the parents are in charge and parent–child relationships are not relationships among equals. The goal is to create a calm environment for the patient and family to address issues. If the family is avoidant of the primary issues, this format will have a higher likelihood of engendering success in catalyzing improved communication habits.

The family session format starts with a review of the ground rules for the session. The suggested ground rules are:

- Your parents are in charge, and there will be no revolution in this session.

---

[17] The roadblocks may be typical resistance that family systems put up to maintain equilibrium.

- I do not live in your house(s), I do not see what actually goes on, and I cannot be the judge in "he said/she said" situations.
- This is a problem-solving session. You have problems. I assume you want things to be better, and we will look for solutions.
- I am going to get a list from each of you what we are going to talk about. We will talk through the list and when we are done . . . we are done . . . we leave the room.

After stating the ground rules, the clinician should poll the participants to create the list on paper, noting who had what concerns. The clinician should start with asking the parents what their concerns are. The clinician can proceed in age order of the other participants or go around the room. If a participant is stumped about what to put on the list, the clinician should move to the next person and give second chances before diving into the list of problems.

It helps to start logically at the top of the list. If there are any similar issues, the clinician can bundle them together.[18] The participant originating the concern should be the first to elaborate on it. The clinician has a choice of whether to go in a wheel-spoke fashion as in a group or simply prompt the participants in general to respond. A good standard to follow is that each participant be given a chance to give feedback on an issue.

Steering a family session in a solution-focused direction requires attending to the problem-focused interaction and reflecting back to the family behaviors and situations that can be changed. An appropriate reflection may be the clinician's observation that the discussion is not headed in a solution-focused direction. On the other hand, the clinician may ask questions of the participants as to what is needed. Sometimes the clinician may need to suggest options that the patient and family can choose to try.

Family sessions can go on too long. Family therapy, like all other psychotherapies, can be tiring and stressful.[19] Although emotions can stimulate the production of adrenalin and heightened energy, the clinician, patients, and families all get mentally tired and the family session

---

[18] Discussing similar concerns separately may unnecessarily lengthen the session and be a source of irritation for family members.

[19] It can be a helpful side intervention for the clinician to verbalize that therapy is hard work and everyone seems to be getting tired and that it is normal for everyone to be tired.

stops being productive. It is in the interest of all if the clinician can keep the discussion moving and end the session when the bottom of the list is reached. The clinician can ask if there is anything else to be discussed, but in longer sessions, the patient and family are probably ready to conclude some time before the end of the list is reached.[20]

SCHOOL

School is an element of the PHP level of care but not the IOP level of care. Typically, a school district and hospital or mental health agency set up a classroom as a cooperative venture to provide compulsory education within the applicable laws. The classroom is typically a special-needs class that is legally subject to size limits.

The treatment value of the school setting varies from case to case. For patients with attention-deficit issues, the school is an opportunity to monitor medication compliance and effectiveness. In many school-refusal cases, the program classroom provides an opportunity to clarify whether a case involves an anxiety issue or a behavior/family dysfunction issue. It is also an opportunity for behavior-disordered patients to make an effort to change behaviors.

The commitment and involvement of the teachers and resident school officials have implications for effectiveness. Clinicians should routinely communicate clinical issues and significant events with the teachers. The teachers are experts in educational matters and can offer valuable feedback as to a patient's situation, condition, and future educational needs.[21] The teachers should be considered de facto members of the treatment team.

A lack of cooperation between teachers and clinicians/clinical staff will mutually undermine the other's efforts and ultimately the program milieu. Noncommunicative teachers and program staff tend to be split by manipulative patients. A teacher can inadvertently take away an

---

[20] It is likely that the patient and parent(s) have discussed many of the problems previously and that the participants are putting on a masquerade for the therapist. In emotionally immature and chaotic families, the patient may be trying to use the clinician and the session as tools of manipulation.

[21] Teachers may have access to the patient's computerized school record and provide clinical information on history and status.

incentive being used by a clinician in the cases of children and preteens. It is important that the clinician seek to build and maintain relationships with the teachers to enhance the therapeutic value of the program.

GROUP THERAPY AND PSYCHOEDUCATION

As discussed in Chapter 6, group therapy has different therapeutic values and functions across the different cohorts, but the consistent role of the clinician is to monitor the patients for safety and symptomology. Although what is therapeutic for the different cohorts needs to be a cumulative product of the needs of the patients, it can be generally assumed that:

- Child groups are good for socialization, expression of feelings, and the development of basic coping skills.
- Adolescent and preadolescent groups vary in productivity based on the acuity, cognitive capabilities, and maturity levels of the patients. Not all cohorts are capable of equally benefitting from group therapy.

Psychoeducation for the cohorts will vary based on cognitive abilities. The child cohort may need education on simple social skills, personal safety, and good basic health habits. Because of the dynamics of maturity, self-control, and cognitive levels, the preteen and adolescent cohorts will fluctuate in what is appropriate and educational for the group.[22]

Psychoeducation and group therapy have a blurred boundary in the preteen and adolescent cohorts. Some productive therapy groups can be educationally focused and center around the discussion of topics or concepts. Based on the cumulative immaturity of the milieu and group, the majority of patients may lack the ego skills and motivation to self-disclose in a spontaneous fashion, and the clinician may need to guide the group interaction through the use of subject matter[23] or media such as movie clips or songs. Art therapy can also be an intensely powerful medium used to express feelings and concerns in patients with lower functioning.

---

[22] This discussion avoids suggesting specific topics as it is more crucial for the clinician and team to agree on them.

[23] Fortunately, numerous group materials for children and adolescents have been available on the market for decades and are readily available with the major online booksellers.

The intent of the educational approach in group therapy is to introduce issues and facilitate a common experience in which the patients gain some kind of therapeutic experience.

The larger challenge of groups in the child and adolescent cohort is minimizing disruption by behavior-disordered patients. Group therapy generally assumes that all participants are motivated to talk and to give feedback. However, behavior-disordered patients tend to display apathy and impulsively to externalize discomfort and irritability without empathic insight, thus disrupting the treatment of other patients. Some of these behavior-disordered patients are verbally aggressive, intimidating, and terroristic toward others. They instigate conflict with other behavior-disordered patients. These patients complain that they are bored. Some behavior-disordered patients simply go to sleep in group therapy, which means that the patient is not being disruptive, but the program cannot bill for the patient when revenue is based on a fee versus a per diem basis.

If there is a heavy prevalence of behavior-disordered patients, the clinician is significantly challenged to have any semblance of a group therapy experience. Such groups are frustrating and tend to be chaotic, because a plurality is either impulsive or uninterested in participating in a therapeutic group experience. Such groups may have a large number of patients who may want to talk about the legalization and glorification of drug use. If the clinician is new to the group, he or she may be personally attacked by oppositional and aggressive patients who may be just having some "fun" with the clinician out of boredom. Some clinicians may feel that they can roll with the behavior-disordered patients and keep trying to get a group discussion going, but other clinicians may feel they have to remove disruptive members from the group for a time-out. The clinician and the team should agree on a consistent approach as to how to deal with these situations, such as removing patients from the group or imposing other consequences.

Depending on census, space, and clinician availability, an alternative strategy is to split the cohort according to homogeneous characteristics such as gender, age, or maturity. One example is creating two therapy groups when it is evidenced that the males in the program have a prevalence of ADHD and behavior disorders, whereas the female patients are mature and have a prevalence of depressive disorders. Another example is when half of the patients are immature and younger than 14, and the other half is mature and 16 or older. Patients who appear to have significant conflict or who feed into each other may also be separated.

With this strategy, group topics and approaches can be chosen that result in a group that has a greater likelihood of meeting clinical needs of all patients in this cohort.

DISCHARGE PLANNING

Discharge planning in the child/adolescent cohort has different challenges than those seen in the adult cohorts. There tend to be fewer options for aftercare than for adult patients, particularly in the supply of child psychiatrists. The attending psychiatrist may not necessarily make a specific order for aftercare, which puts the decision in the clinician's lap to review options with the parent. The parent or guardian may not like the available options. Third, it is a job expectation of the clinician to make aftercare appointments, regardless of the parent's or guardian's level of commitment to follow up for the patient.

This aftercare predicament can make the clinician appear as passive-aggressive when it comes to asserting aftercare plans. A way to minimize the aftercare dilemma is to discuss aftercare at admission with the parent(s) or guardian. The clinician's stance should be an appeal to structure and an elaboration of the aftercare expectations.

A UNIQUE PROBLEM: THE MILIEU

The staff can bring negative externalities of poor emotional intelligence and emotional baggage to the child–adolescent milieu. This milieu requires the staff to be mature and to set firm but quiet boundaries with patients. It also requires the staff members to maintain their objectivity about the oppositional defiance of patients and neither personalize it nor engage in countertransference. The structure of a successful milieu must take into account emotional boundaries, the maintenance of which requires the support and cooperation of the full staff.

A staff member's evident emotion or loud speaking voice can agitate a milieu and detract from treatment focus, and this is especially true for the child–adolescent PHP/IOP. Staff horseplay can inadvertently give license to patients to engage in horseplay and teasing that escalate into aggression due to impulsivity and poor anger management. Higher voice volume of staff members tends to agitate patients. Yelling or losing control of their emotions undermines staff members' credibility and emotional control in a unit.[24] Staff members arguing with oppositional patients causes power struggles with the patients that unintentionally reward the patient with negative attention. The patient's negative behavior is inadvertently reinforced. The patient is motivated to continue testing limits, which reenacts the enmeshed parent–child boundaries at home.[25] Staff members can unwittingly escalate the anxiety and tension of milieus with their own anxious, tense overreactions and arguments with patients.

The agitation and tension of the child and adolescent milieu can accumulate and intensify at the unit's nursing station. The nursing station is a central location that draws oppositional and attention-seeking patients. Depending on the point in time of the program schedule, oppositional and defiant patients can cause more milieu disruption with an audience at or near the nursing station.

Another unique challenge of the milieu is seen when patients and their families demand special treatment. This most often centers around food.[26] Some families also demand that patients continue with their outpatient therapists at the same time as being in the program.[27] The parents of these families may call frequently throughout the day with concerns or demands. The parent may instigate drama in the form of complaints about the psychiatrist or clinician. If the staff sets limits with the parent, the parent may in turn complain to the supervisor about the staff being rude,

---

[24] Staff members yelling at patients could constitute abuse.

[25] Transactional analysis (Berne, 1964/2004) is a useful conceptual framework for this issue. Oppositional defiant children and adolescents are essentially conditioned at home that they can argue. They have learned how to cross emotional boundaries with parents and will make adult-like and personal criticisms of staff members. If a staff member is not mindful of the dynamics of this exchange, the patient may continue using this newly discovered power and target the staff member with further personal attacks.

[26] Eating-disordered patients may have imposed diets requiring food brought from home. Furthermore, picky eaters may have control issues that are part of the family system problem. Limits should be set with the patient and family that any food the patients eat in the program will be provided by the program or hospital kitchen in accordance with any and all accreditation standards.

[27] In this problem, the patient can split the outpatient therapist, parents, and the program staff.

insensitive, or condescending.[28] When such demands are acquiesced to, the family and/or patient dictate treatment and potentially disrupt the milieu.

CONCLUSIONS

This chapter discussed the distinct problems and challenges of the child and adolescent PHP/IOP cohort. It reviewed the patient subcohorts with their different development levels and treatment needs. It covered some of the challenges of the behavior-disordered patient and the different treatment modalities and distinctions found in this milieu. Success for the clinician and staff in the child–adolescent PHP/IOP cohort will likely be manifested more by the absence of problems than the rate of positive treatment outcomes.

Mindfulness of reasonable expectations is crucial when evaluating success in this PHP/IOP cohort. This cohort has more extraneous family variables that determine whether treatment is even going to address the presenting problems. A family must have the resources and commitment to participate in treatment. When parents are low functioning themselves, they are not necessarily aware or honest about their contributions to the problems. The patient is still in the family setting outside of program hours, and if the family is not making the necessary changes, the PHP/IOP will unlikely be an effective intervention.

Furthermore, social and legal systems tend to refer children and adolescents to the PHP/IOP as an available intervention for a problem that actually is not shown to be a psychiatric problem or is only a part of a psychiatric problem. Parents and guardians present with the hope that treatment will rescue them from legal consequences. A child's or adolescent's treatment compliance and attendance in the PHP/IOP is a function of the parent's level of control and influence, and frequent absences tend to indicate that the parent is not in control and had likely lost control a long time before treatment began. Because the PHP/IOP is limited in these cases, it is a symbolic "rule out" that psychiatric issues are not the problem.

REFERENCE

Berne, E. (2004). *Games people play*. New York, NY: Ballantine Books. (Original work published 1964).

---

[28] These complaints are nebulous and emotional and may have a modicum of fact.

CHAPTER THIRTEEN

CHEMICAL DEPENDENCY/ CO-OCCURRING DISORDERS

The chemical dependency (CD)[1] PHP/IOP is a specialized form of outpatient treatment that aims to help an addicted patient cease the use of his or her substance of choice, whether alcohol or illicit substances. The typical patient meeting the criteria for admission has a maladaptive pattern of alcohol or substance use that has caused some functional impairment and risk. The typical clinician working with this cohort is either a credentialed alcohol and drug counselor or a clinician who has significant experience with this population.[2] The overall goal in most treatment approaches is for the patient to start and continue to be abstinent.

Due to managed care pressure, CD treatment at the PHP/IOP level has replaced the inpatient and residential levels as the first choice of treatment in many alcohol and substance abuse cases (Washton, 1997). Inpatient treatment tends to be reserved for patients who have an immediate risk of severe and life-threatening withdrawal or a co-occurring condition of suicidal ideation with a plan or an inability to contract for safety.

This chapter discusses some of the unique challenges presented by the treatment of patients with CD and co-occurring disorders at the PHP and IOP level of care. Although it describes programming at this level,

---

[1] The term *chemical dependency* is used in this chapter as opposed to *addiction*, *substance use*, or *substance abuse*. There have been a number of fads regarding the terms used to refer to addiction over the years. Therefore, the use of the term *chemical dependency* is a stylistic choice.

[2] Many such credentialed clinicians are in recovery themselves.

it does not discuss substance abuse counseling techniques but rather describes the application of the different games to be played.[3]

PROGRAMMING DESCRIPTION

This section provides background on CD treatment at the PHP/IOP level of care. It discusses typical patient profiles, expectations, and programming structure.

As with other cohorts, the PHP level of care typically has patients with greater symptom severity than those patients found in the IOP. The PHP patient may be a step-down from inpatient status or a direct admission. Regardless, the PHP patient has psychiatric issues severe enough to mandate treatment be a priority over a sole focus on sobriety.

The IOP-level patient in this cohort typically does not have psychiatric issues. The patient is typically focused solely on abstinence and recovery, and programming can occur in the evening when the services of a psychiatrist are not needed.[4]

The patient who is a working adult typically has an expected treatment outcome of ceasing use and maintaining abstinence in accordance with employer requirements. The patient referred by an employer or employee assistance program (EAP) provider may have additional drug testing and treatment requirements for returning to work in order to maintain his or her employment status. The specific expectations placed on this patient vary according to professional standards and work situations.[5]

---

[3] The Substance Abuse and Mental Health Services Administration published a series of treatment improvement protocols (TIPS), including a volume on intensive outpatient treatment (SAMHSA, 2006). This volume is available in hardcopy and online in portable document format (PDF). The reader is referred to this source as a comprehensive guide.

[4] A possible challenge is that staffing an evening program may be difficult because the work hours are unattractive for clinicians.

[5] The stringency of expectation depends on security issues, safety issues, and professional standard issues. For example, nurses, heavy equipment operators, and individuals working in high-security situations may have more stringent requirements than clerical or customer service employees.

Many patients not referred by an employer may be referred by the legal system due to an arrest for driving while under the influence, a drug charge, or for a probation violation such as a positive drug screen. Many adolescent patients fit into this category. The patients referred by the legal system are usually expected to provide proof of treatment compliance or face greater consequences such as incarceration.

The nonworking adult on disability admitted to the PHP/IOP for chemical dependency treatment may have been involved in a disruptive situation or an event that precipitated treatment. The patient may also have a legal issue or may have been using substances to the point of spending all of his or her money and then began to go through life-threatening withdrawal. The patient may have had a psychiatric inpatient admission where it was determined that substance use was both a precipitant and a problem. The patient may have a serious and persistent mental illness that is exacerbated by the patient's substance use. The patient may have had an ultimatum to get treated or get kicked out of his or her residence. The essential reality in these cases is that the patient needs to stop chemical/substance usage and to be stable or face further life consequences as a result of the substance use.

The course of treatment in the CD cohort involves group therapy, education, and homework. A psychiatrist may supervise medical withdrawal issues and prescribe appropriate psychiatric medications.[6] Group therapy is much like other PHP/IOP group sessions, but the focus tends to be on (a) feelings as they pertain to the patient's relapse challenges and (b) coping strategies to avoid relapse. The education sessions may contain information about coping skills but will tend to focus on addiction, recovery, and relapse. The homework may include proprietary material or the completion of the first and second steps and reading chapters from the pertinent 12-step "big book." Some of the homework may include the patient going to 12-step meetings, identifying a temporary sponsor, and bringing back proof of this support group attendance. Case management/treatment planning tends to focus on patient accountability with the homework and urine drug screens.[7] A program may offer a

---

[6] The regimen could be a psychiatric medication for symptomology or a medicine that either blocks effects or discourages use.

[7] Alcohol is not picked up by urine drug screens. Some programs may use a breathalyzer to monitor abstinence when alcohol is the drug of choice.

weekly family group and an ongoing aftercare group of limited duration.[8] A typical treatment outcome of the CD-PHP/IOP is that a patient will have complied with attendance, done the homework, and maintained abstinence as evidenced by clean drug screens.

There are patients in the various age cohorts who may show both CD and psychiatric symptoms.[9] The substance and alcohol use may be a cause or precipitant for recurrence of symptoms or readmission to inpatient care. On the other hand, the patient may be using illicit substances and alcohol as a maladaptive medication for the psychiatric symptoms. Assessment and treatment includes determining whether a patient's symptoms are primarily organic psychiatric issues or caused by alcohol and/or drug use.

Since the 1990s, there has been a focus on integrating psychiatric and CD treatment as championed in large part by the U.S. government through SAMHSA (SAMHSA, 2006) and its spearheading and funding of research.[10] The terms used to describe this integration are *dual diagnosis* and *co-occurring*. SAMHSA has printed substantive professional and informational materials on CD, mental health, and co-occurring issues. These materials are in the public domain and are available on its website (www.samhsa.gov).[11]

Co-occurring treatment is the simultaneous or integrated treatment of mental health and CD issues. The goals are for the patient to demonstrate symptom stability, abstinence, and connection to a sober support system. For the PHP/IOP setting, it can mean the creation of a subcohort of patients simultaneously dealing with both psychiatric and CD issues or splitting treatment time for a patient between CD and psychiatric therapy groups.

---

[8] The family group and aftercare group are often conditions of a managed care organization (MCO) contract.

[9] There are two basic patterns of co-occurring disorders. Patients can show depressive symptoms from using alcohol, marijuana, and cocaine. A person using cocaine can have suicidal ideation. On the other hand, a patient with schizophrenia or bipolar disorder may be drinking alcohol or using substances instead of taking appropriate psychiatric medication. The general result of both patterns is presentation for treatment.

[10] A key term connected with much of CD and co-occurring treatment is *evidence based*, which refers to having evaluative research supporting a treatment approach's effectiveness.

[11] The materials may be available in hardcopy, PDF, and html format.

CHALLENGES

As described in this section, the challenges for CD and co-occurring treatment at the PHP/IOP level are financial, milieu related, and psychiatric in nature. The financial issues have to do with the cost of treatment resources and managed care constraints. The milieu issues are related to the blending of patients in and out of the program. The psychiatric issues may involve the underestimation of the symptom severity of some patients. The discharge challenges are an issue when a patient is expected to be in treatment as an expectation of maintaining employment.

The financial challenges are usually (a) the managed care pressure through utilization management to shorten treatment time and (b) the fact that many educational resources are proprietary in nature. [12] As discussed in previous chapters, MCOs offer limited time for patients to be in treatment and expect completion of the treatment tasks within that time. [13] A clinician must demonstrate substantial clinical reasons for the extension of a patient's treatment. Furthermore, the CD field is rich with educational resources that are proprietary and require specific training and an ongoing usage fee that may be financially prohibitive to the organization. [14] The inability to purchase the proprietary education materials may place an onus on the staff to create appropriate educational material about addiction, recovery, and relapse prevention that are relevant to the specific age population. Furthermore, the staff will have to press patients to engage in the desired treatment homework and support group attendance within the number of covered days as allowed by the MCO.

The patient milieu may be a challenge in that often patients are encouraged to attend 12-step groups outside of the regular program hours. There is a high likelihood that patients will go to some of the same

---

[12] Public insurance such as Medicare and Medicaid have limits to group size, which in turn impose fiscal constraints.

[13] Copayment for CD-IOP services are sometimes cost prohibitive for patients.

[14] Many programs advertise that they use certain proprietary material. In these cases, it can be assumed that (a) the clinician(s) have been through the official training, (b) the organization pays the yearly usage fee, and (c) the clinician and organization maintain fidelity with the proprietary program design. Some of these proprietary programs include Matrix, Seven Challenges, Recovery Dynamics, and Prime for Life.

12-step groups and make extraneous connections. With these connec-tions, cliques and shadow groups may form and cause undercurrents to occur in the program inciting patients to distract each other from treat-ment focus.

A third challenge concerns underlying psychiatric issues. Some higher functioning patients with co-occurring disorders may not be inter-ested in addressing psychiatric issues and may be hiding suicidal ide-ations behind alcohol and drug use. A person with bipolar disorder may disrupt a group session with impulsive and manic behavior. An adoles-cent with attention deficit hyperactivity disorder (ADHD) who is non-medicated may be attention seeking and engaging in clowning.[15] A larger issue may be the presence of personality-disordered patients who create disruption in the program through openly and personally challenging a clinician and instigating staff splitting and drama.

Personality-disordered patients are often screened from group ther-apy in the outpatient setting but are not necessarily screened from the PHP/IOP setting.[16] The patient with a personality disorder may be disruptive through monopolization, angry outbursts, and drama in the group ses-sions. The patient may demonstrate noncompliance in the homework and attendance, suggesting an incapability to engage in the necessary but emo-tionally painful reflection on relapse triggers because of a lack of inner or ego strength.[17] A personality-disordered patient may have a cycle of multi-ple readmissions after administrative discharges due to absenteeism.

Somewhat related to the aforementioned challenge, many work-ing patients have specific expectations from employers and an EAP. In a sense, the patient has the ultimate responsibility of compliance with

---

[15] A medication-compliant adolescent with ADHD may still be disruptive in an afternoon IOP because the medication has metabolized out of his or her system.

[16] A psychiatrist discharging a patient from inpatient care may determine that a patient's personality disorder issues are such that he or she will not benefit from PHP or IOP treatment.

[17] A colloquial term that refers to this situation is *two-stepping*, which means the individual can do the first two steps of a 12-step program but is unable to cope with admitting powerlessness and is unable to deal with the emotions, guilt, and shame faced in the third, fourth, and fifth steps. Such an individual may relapse or be what is called a "dry drunk," which refers to someone who is otherwise a difficult or unpleasant person who is not demonstrating serenity.

these expectations. This challenge can get complicated, in that the EAP may be a referral source that the program depends on for new patients. As discussed in Chapter 5, there is the risk of the instigation of drama based on an EAP provider's degree of involvement and the level of the patient's honesty and cooperation in the treatment process. Furthermore, the EAP provider may place extra treatment requirements on the patient that either the patient does not understand or that contradict the program design.[18] Depending on how depressed or impaired the patient is in terms of detoxification symptoms, the clinician may have to assess the situation and advocate for the patient to ensure that he or she understands his or her requirements to return to work.

APPLICATIONS OF THE GAMES

Many of the basic games already discussed in this book apply to the routines of the CD-IOP setting. The games used in the therapeutic milieu, treatment planning, group therapy, psychoeducation,[19] and safety should be applicable and useful for the CD-IOP clinician to deal with the previously described challenges and to successfully organize practice activities.

The larger of the challenges faced tend to concern the time constraint placed on patients by managed care. As discussed in Chapter 4, a patient with managed care insurance will be given a limited amount of time to be in treatment. This can put a squeeze on the working patient having to comply with an EAP provider's directives.[20] In response to this squeeze, the clinician will likely need to construct a script for a patient in

---

[18] If the EAP provider is a significant referral source, there is a tendency to acquiesce to whatever demands the provider may make, so that more referrals are made. The demands may cross boundaries, as some EAP providers may seem to dictate treatment to clinicians.

[19] Financial constraints may also prohibit some programs from purchasing and supplying patients' copies of the Alcoholics Anonymous (AA) or Narcotics Anonymous (NA) big book (Alcoholic Anonymous, 2001; Narcotics Anonymous, 2008).

[20] Such directives may include proof of the 12-step meeting attendance, documentation of clean drug screens, and a letter of compliance from a psychiatrist or therapist.

this situation.[21] Such a script will guide the patient in a timeline fashion as to what needs to be done to be discharged and in communicating the MCO constraints to the EAP provider.

Addressing the challenge of psychiatric issues in a substance abuse setting is open to multiple interpretations. Because it is usually not possible to screen patients for appropriateness for group therapy prior to admission, adjustments in group composition may be necessary. When it is not possible to form co-occurring groups, there are at least four clarifying questions used to decide whether the patient with co-occurring issues should be referred to CD over psychiatric treatment:

- Is there a psychiatric impairment that inhibits or renders the patient incapable of focusing on abstinence and recovery?
- What is the group composition of the rest of the CD-IOP group?
- Is this patient disruptive to the milieu of the program?
- Is the patient with co-occurring issues sufficiently motivated and capable enough to engage in the necessary recovery homework?

If a patient turns out to have a significant psychiatric impairment and the rest of the group does not, it may be in the interest of both the patient and the group that the patient be referred to a different group. A patient with significant psychiatric symptomology such as mania or florid psychosis can be disruptive in a CD group on account of the patient's impulsivity and bizarre thought content.[22] In such situations, the symptomatic patient should be considered for an appropriate psychiatric group and the CD issues should be processed as individual treatment goals.

Furthermore, there is a question as to whether a patient with co-occurring issues is sufficiently motivated for recovery and capable of participating in CD treatment. A patient with significant psychiatric issues may be too manic, too depressed, or too anxious to be focused on recovery activities such as going to meetings. A patient with bipolar disorder or a personality disorder may have to be referred to a psychiatric

---

[21] These scripts should be possible to make if there are a limited number of EAP providers that have recurring contact with the program.

[22] A patient with disruptive psychiatric symptoms can inadvertently scare other patients away through tangents in the group or emotional and threatening outbursts.

PHP/IOP group or referred to outpatient CD therapy if unable to handle the intensity of the program or is disruptive to the group.

Some of the clinician's prerogative may be precluded by a psychiatrist, but when a psychiatrist is not involved, decisions should be based on a principled balance between the needs of the group and the needs of a patient.[23] A patient with co-occurring issues should be stable and have a sufficient level of function to be capable of handling the stress of abstinence and the focus on recovery, which requires potentially painful reflection.

CONCLUSIONS

This chapter briefly described the treatment of patients with CD and co-occurring disorders at the PHP and IOP level of care. It avoided discussion of CD-specific techniques but reviewed setting-specific challenges and corresponding strategies.

There are several finance-related challenges for this population. The increasing prevalence of managed care in both public and private insurance means shorter patient stays. There are a number of proprietary treatment approaches that are highly touted but require expensive certification, patient materials, and yearly franchising fees; these may be cost prohibitive, and, as a result, clinicians may have to create educational materials. The clinician and program staff may need to address these challenges creatively so as effectively guide the patient to meet as many treatment goals as reasonably possible within the time limits.

Although the program milieu may be a challenge, the co-occurring disorder movement is opening up challenges in terms of addressing the needs of patients with both psychiatric and CD issues. Some patients with disruptive psychiatric symptoms are a challenge for CD counselors

---

[23] A clinician also needs to evaluate whether he or she is competent to handle the co-occurring patient's case. A psychiatric clinician should seek supervision or consultation when the patient's CD issues manifest as more severe than disclosed in the admission assessment. On the other hand, the CD counselor should also seek supervision or consultation when a patient's psychiatric issues such as anxiety, mania, suicidality, or personality disorder are disruptive or beyond the counselor's knowledge and experience.

who have little previous mental health experience. The creation of homogeneous groups is one solution for the disruptive patient, but it may not be possible based on available resources; the use of a decision-making protocol may be necessary in the interest of balancing patient and group needs.

The involvement of an EAP provider may create some challenges given that the provider has power as a referral source. Some EAP providers may insist on being involved in treatment and may continue to communicate with patients throughout the course of treatment. The EAP provider may have to be addressed with tact and diplomacy, and the EAP expectations should be integrated when possible into the treatment.

CD treatment at the PHP/IOP level can be an efficient and effective community-based form of treatment in which the patient intensely focuses on abstinence and sobriety in the face of relapse triggers. Attention to the challenges and strategies is crucial for clinician and program success.

REFERENCES

Alcoholics Anonymous. (2001). *Alcoholics Anonymous* (4th ed.). New York, NY: A. A. World Services.

Center for Substance Abuse Treatment, Substance Abuse and Mental Health Services Administration (SAMHSA). (2006). *Substance abuse: Clinical issues in intensive outpatient treatment. Treatment Improvement Protocol (TIP) Series 47* (DHHS Publication No. SMA 06-4182). Retrieved from http://www.ncbi.nlm.nih.gov/books/NBK64093/pdf/TOC.pdf

Narcotics Anonymous. (2008). *Narcotics Anonymous* (6th ed.). Chatsworth, CA: Narcotics Anonymous World Services.

Washton, A. M. (1997). Evolution of intensive outpatient treatment (IOP) as a "legitimate" treatment modality for chemical dependency. In E. Gottheil & B. Stimmel (Eds.), *Intensive outpatient treatment for the addictions* (pp. xix–xxv). New York, NY: Haworth Press.

Chapter Fourteen

The Borderline Personality– Disordered Patient[1]

*H*aving a personality-disordered patient or dealing with a patient's personality-disordered family member is inevitable in any clinical setting. The successful clinician with longevity in the field has learned through trial and error to develop the skills needed to identify and successfully work with personality-disordered individuals. Although they have a low prevalence in the general population, personality-disordered individuals have a high prevalence in treatment settings.[2] The prevalence comparisons point to the reality that treatment settings are collection nodes for individuals with personality disorders.

Borderline personality disorder has been the subject of thousands of publications and remains a source of contention and controversy as to its cause and appropriate treatments. There are studies on both group and individual therapies as being effective treatments for individuals with borderline personality. Regardless of the approach, it is generally agreed that patients with borderline personality disorder ("borderline patients") are difficult persons to interact with and to treat.

---

[1] This chapter assumes that the reader has an understanding of borderline personality disorder. It does not go into an explanation or discussion of its etiology or symptomology.

[2] Lenzenweger, Lane, Loranger, and Kessler (2007) identified a 6.0% prevalence rate of cluster B personality disorders in the National Comorbidity Study. There is no specific epidemiological research about what presents in partial hospitalization program/intensive outpatient program settings. It is hypothesized here that there will be more narcissistic traits presenting in the child/adolescent cohort because those patients typically have little to no choice in agreeing to treatment. However, it is hypothesized that female patients with borderline personality will be more prevalent than male patients with borderline personality in line with existing epidemiological findings.

As discussed in previous chapters, a partial hospitalization program (PHP)/intensive outpatient program (IOP) will likely get various personality-disordered patients without warning. The patients are admitted because they meet specific criteria of acuity and not because of the personality-disorder symptoms. The clinician and staff will not always recognize that a patient has a personality disorder until a problem occurs.

In the PHP/IOP setting, the borderline personality could belong to the patient, the parent, or both. In the adult cohorts, the clinician will typically see the borderline personality in the patient. In the child/adolescent[3] cohort, the clinician may be dealing with a child with borderline traits[4], a parent with borderline traits, or a combination of both. Dealing with a parent with borderline personality adds complexity to the treatment as the parent can undermine addressing the patient's salient issues. Similar to the adult PHP/IOP setting, there is no warning that a child or adolescent's parent has borderline personality unless there is familiarity with the parent prior to the patient's admission (or readmission).

Patients with borderline personality disorder tend to be taxing on the clinician and staff due to disruptive behavior and suicidality. Some of these behaviors include:

- Mood swings and anger outbursts
- Poor boundaries of intruding into the personal affairs of other patients, the clinician, and staff[5]
- Competing for attention with embellished and perfidious tales that paint the patient as having suffered more than others
- Repeatedly disclosing dramatic stories of making a suicide attempt a few days after the fact[6]

---

[3] The child of a borderline personality may have the traits of a different personality disorder such as a narcissistic personality.

[4] A person is not supposed to be diagnosed with a personality disorder until age 18; for the duration of the chapter, the word "traits" is omitted when discussing adolescents and children.

[5] The borderline patient may make an unsolicited criticism of a staff member or another patient. How the staff member responds to the patient determines how much power the patient will gain.

[6] Usually the patient will not be suicidal at the time of the disclosure. The patient often has a tone of anger that may insinuate the clinician incompetently missed something.

These patients can be risky and dangerous to the point of physical aggression, but more commonly use verbal aggression and distorted but serious allegations against the clinician and staff.

The children of borderline personalities often end up in treatment due to parental dysfunction, abuse, and emotional neglect. A parent with borderline personality disorder tends to lack the distress tolerance required to manage a child with attention deficit hyperactivity disorder (ADHD) and labels the child as an uncontrollable behavior problem. A parent with borderline personality disorder may portray an angry teenager as out of control when the patient's behavior is shown to be a natural response to the parent's smothering control and emotional abuse.[7] Some patients present as possible cases of Munchhausen's syndrome by proxy in which the parent with borderline personality disorder appears to make the child mentally ill.[8] In all these cases, the borderline personality–disordered parent wants the child fixed, but does not accept responsibility for any part of the problem.

This chapter discusses a suggested game of working with borderline personality disorders in the PHP/IOP setting. It reviews the challenges of working with the borderline personality patient and parent. It does not discuss the etiology of borderline personality disorder or a prescribed, alternative course of psychotherapy, but offers some cues for recognizing borderline personality, suggests practice strategies using the other games discussed in this book, and suggests ways to minimize disruption in the PHP/IOP setting.[9]

---

[7] This could be an etiology for eating disorders. Some of these children are looking for some sense of control.

[8] In the Munchausen's by proxy cases, there is an abuse of power. The parent is extremely controlling and has no insight into his or her contribution to the problem. Any rebellion by the child or adolescent gets defined as mental illness by the parent. The child or adolescent may have a history of multiple psychiatric admissions due to suicidal ideation and possible attempts. The parent will likely say that none of the prior treatment episodes have helped. There may have been at least one child protective services referral for abuse of the treatment system.

[9] The existing treatment modalities should be sufficient. If the patient needs something different, then he or she should be referred to the appropriate program when available.

CHALLENGES

This section describes some of the predominant challenges of the borderline patient in the PHP/IOP setting. It discusses the individual, group, family, and milieu issues that exist when the borderline personality belongs to the patient, and the family issues that arise when the borderline personality appears in the parent. It suggests these challenges in general trends.

Treatment Savvy and Help Rejection in Case Management and Individual Therapy[10]

In terms of the individual challenges, whether in treatment planning or individual therapy, many borderline patients are treatment savvy but claim that nothing yet has helped their problems. Many of these patients have had numerous treatment episodes and will demonstrate detailed knowledge of coping skills and theory but disqualify suggested coping skills and techniques. The clinician often struggles with the patient in trying to identify goals.

When the borderline patient does identify goals, they tend to be unrealistic and nebulous. If the clinician attempts to focus the patient, an argument may ensue with the patient refusing to commit to reasonable and attainable goals. The resulting struggle between the clinician and patient can devolve to the patient claiming to be a victim of the clinician. A severe outcome of such a struggle results when this patient verbally attacks the clinician face to face in an attempt to turn the tables regarding treatment planning.[11]

Some borderline patients display sexualized behaviors and focus on sexual issues in treatment planning when the clinician is of the opposite sex. The patient may provocatively claim that the main problem is

---

[10] Depending on the payer source and program design, the meeting with the patient is going to be a case management session or an individual therapy session. In the adult cohorts with Medicare as a core payer source, the individual meeting will be case management, which discusses treatment needs, progress, and goals. In the child and adolescent cohort with Medicaid as the core payer source, the individual session will be individual psychotherapy.

[11] The attack could be the patient claiming that the clinician does not understand or is pushing too hard.

hypersexuality.[12] When the clinician works to set limits about sexual issues, the patient may try to turn tables or cross boundaries by asking whether the clinician has a personal problem with sex. By doing so, a borderline patient may try to usurp power within the therapeutic relationship. A clinician may struggle with giving the patient an answer that is not an accidental disclosure of inappropriate personal information.

Another challenge in treatment planning and individual therapy for the borderline patient is the patient's failure to comply with agreed-upon homework in accordance with the goals. The patient may have no explanation for failure to comply. He or she can get into a power struggle and instigate drama with a clinician and will claim victimhood when the clinician demonstrates anger in the form of frustration.[13]

The Challenges in Group Therapy

In the group therapy sessions, individuals with borderline personality (sometimes it may be the same patient) play a number of extreme and difficult roles that are challenging for the clinician.[14] These include:

- The raging intimidator who is defiantly hostile and critical of the clinician and other patients in front of the group[15]
- The hopeless attention seeker and debater who claims to be in crisis and asks the group for help but will then reject any suggestion
- The monopolizer who will take up most if not all of the whole group session talking
- The "door knobber" who starts to talk at the end of the group hour and will not stop talking at the scheduled end-time

---

[12] There may actually be a modicum of truth to the borderline-personality patients' disclosure of excessive sexual activity.

[13] The patient may complain that the clinician is expecting too much.

[14] Yalom and Leszcz (2005) note, "One borderline may be markedly dissimilar clinically to each other" (p. 421).

[15] This particular person is unlikely to come back the next day after an outburst. The patient may come back 1 to 2 days later, if at all. This situation is illustrative of the characterological aspect of borderline personality because the complaint is often immature and the personality-disordered individual tends not to have the integrity to confront or complain personally.

- The junior therapist who gives everyone else dogmatic advice while avoiding facing personal issues
- The "insinuator" who gives frequent dirty looks and insinuates self-righteousness through dramatic avoidance gestures toward others, which may include changing seats
- The provocateur who seeks attention through disclosures about suicidality or sexual issues
- The accuser who may actually "confront" the clinician about being mad at a patient in the middle of the group session or in a one-on-one setting after the group session[16]
- The anxious waif who presents as a small child who sits in a fetal position or has to leave the group frequently because of intense anxiety

All of the challenges posed by this type of behavior can degrade the quality of the group experience for other patients, but in turn, the borderline patient can openly disrupt the group in defiance when the clinician attempts to confront or set limits in any one of the previously described situations. The clinician is challenged to respond in such a way that minimizes, if not neutralizes, the effect of the borderline patient in the least disruptive manner.

A different kind of challenge arises when a new clinician substitutes or takes over a group containing more than one borderline personality patient. The borderline patients in the group tend to exhibit abandonment reactions about the loss of the old clinician and displace that anger toward the new clinician. Depending on how fragile the patients' egos are, the emotion they express may come in the form of an angry cabal attacking the new clinician. This situation can be especially taxing when the other program staff and supervisor have low emotional intelligence and become rescuers in the drama instigated by the borderline patient(s).[17]

---

[16] The clinician could say, "So what if I am mad at you?" The patient will likely respond: "I can't stand anyone being mad at me." The clinician could counter, "It sounds like you are feeling very anxious and engaging in a lot of worry. Maybe you can talk about that it in the group?"

[17] Some staff and supervisors may actually present as taking the side of the complaining patients in these cases, casting doubt about the new clinician's competence.

The Challenge in the Family Session

The borderline personality in the family session tends to avoid being dialectical in addressing issues and seeking solutions. The child with borderline traits may have chaotic enmeshment with the parents as evidenced by an inappropriate bargaining position and stonewalling of the discussion of salient issues. The borderline patient may manipulatively threaten suicidality based on his or her assumptions of family members' thoughts and feelings.[18] Family members may report exasperation, resentment, and burnout over the patient's behaviors. The patient may personally attack the clinician or a parent to avoid talking about issues. The clinician has the challenge of conducting a meaningful and orderly family session that furthers the treatment plan.

The Interpersonal Challenge in the Milieu

The typical PHP/IOP setting is an acute milieu where the borderline personality patient's dysfunctional behavior can manifest beyond the therapy and treatment planning sessions. The reality of working with the borderline personality in this setting is that the borderline personality is still the borderline personality. Although treatment may help a borderline patient learn different or improved coping skills, it will not stop the patient from manifesting maladaptive and dysfunctional social behaviors that impact the milieu through a number of externalities.[19]

This reality of the borderline still being the borderline is significant in both the clinician–patient interactions and in the PHP/IOP milieu. A common feature of a borderline personality is the tendency to seek control without regard for the rights and needs of others. It is all about the patient. The borderline patient tends to have little to no inner regulation for balance, fairness, and order in relationships.[20] Many borderline personalities demonstrate a self-concept of victimhood, which engenders a self-righteous sense of entitlement to control others through whatever means the patient deems necessary.

---

[18] An example of this is the patient with borderline personality disorder saying to other family members "I am going to be suicidal if you exaggerate things."

[19] This use of externality refers to secondary and unexpected effects or consequences.

[20] Not all borderline personalities have this feature.

Some of the borderline patient's control attempts come in the form of complaints about the clinician to other staff and other patients. The patient with borderline personality disorder either will tend to take the self-righteous victim role or will act as a caretaking rescuer motivated by a perceived moral imperative.[21] There may be a germ of validity to the borderline patient's criticism, but the whole of the criticism consists of an embellished husk of nebulous, emotional reasons. Such vague criticism can include the following:

- The clinician does not care.
- The clinician expects too much.
- The clinician seems angry.
- Other patients are uncomfortable with the clinician.
- The clinician does not seem to be listening.
- The clinician lost his or her temper with the patient or told the patient to shut up.[22]

Most of these complaints can evolve into drama based on staff reaction.

The kernel of truth revealed in these interpersonal settings may be undetermined or it may be established that the clinician had set limits or confronted the borderline patient.[23] In making the complaint, the patient omits or embellishes the context and claims to report the feelings of other patients.[24] The borderline patient can cross emotional boundaries when staff react naïvely or emotionally to this patient's criticism and, in turn, join in with the patient in also criticizing the clinician.

There is a probability that the borderline patient's anger, impulsivity, and attention-seeking behaviors will engender disruption in the treatment of other acutely depressed and anxious patients. There is the

---

[21] The complaint is about either how the patient is being treated by the clinician or how the clinician is not treating another patient.

[22] Although this criticism is a demonstration of embellishment, it still is a complaint that will likely have to be investigated, given that most hospitals would classify this as patient abuse. Because of his or her fragile ego, the patient with borderline personality disorder may interpret a firm confrontation as yelling.

[23] A borderline adolescent with a passive parent may fabricate a complaint about a clinician or staff member out of passive-aggressive retaliation for a consequence.

[24] The borderline personality patient may also be projecting a feeling onto the other patients in these situations.

likelihood that the borderline personality patient will expend effort to split and instigate conflict and drama among staff and other patients.

As part of their tendency to have poor boundaries, PHP/IOP patients with borderline personality often become enmeshed to the point of losing treatment focus, which is an inherent liability for the clinician and the organization. As discussed in Chapter 2, enmeshed patients tend to form a shadow group outside of the group.[25] When the clinician attempts to assert limits with the patients about appropriate boundaries and the need to cooperate with the clinician in formal treatment, the patients with borderline personality disorder may revolt and engage in drama, as discussed in the following text.

Extreme anxiety is another challenge seen in patients with borderline personality in the PHP/IOP setting. A patient may state to numerous staff and patients that he or she is worried about others being mad at him or her. An adolescent or adult patient may sit in a fetal position in a chair and refuse to talk in group therapy.[26] A third manifestation in the PHP/IOP milieu is the avoidant borderline personality patient who exhibits poor attendance and agoraphobia.[27] The borderline patients often get discharged for nonattendance or they stop coming as they claim excessive anxiety while refusing to engage in treatment.[28]

Challenges From Within

Clinicians and treatment teams often experience countertransference toward patients with borderline personality disorder. It is normal to

---

[25] In their enmeshment, patients with borderline personality disorder can make each other the primary therapeutic alliance versus the clinician and group. They can refuse to discuss crises appropriately with the clinician and instead rely on each other. The clinician attempting to set limits can present as the villain.

[26] The adolescent with borderline traits also tends to frequently request to leave group therapy or school due to a somatic complaint.

[27] Some adolescents with borderline traits with school refusal and poor program attendance may be enmeshed with a mother with borderline personality disorder.

[28] The borderline personality patient tends to demonstrate that there is a relationship between control and anxiety. He or she may be getting secondary benefits by staying in an extreme anxiety state. Over a short period of time, the patient's secondary benefits do become evident, and when confronted about taking responsibility, the patient may stop coming for treatment without notice.

respond in defensive anger when another individual makes a personal attack. The average clinician has invested time, money, and effort into the education and extra training required to become a clinician and the patient is showing immaturity in making such criticisms. The clinician and clinical staff should practice mindfulness and objectivity about patient attacks and maintain a professional demeanor.

The Borderline Personality Patient in the Parent Role

When the parent with borderline personality disorder ("borderline parent") admits a child or adolescent to a PHP/IOP setting, the clinician may face several complications:[29]

- The borderline parent may enforce patient silence about what goes on in the home. The parent may then interrogate the patient at the end of the program day about what the patient and the clinician discussed.[30]
- The borderline parent may confront the clinician about the clinician's statements or feedback to the patient and call the supervisor to "fire" the clinician.[31]
- The borderline parent may claim that the clinician was offensive or patronizing.
- The borderline parent might be avoidant of family sessions after admission.
- When the borderline parent comes to the family session, he or she will likely be argumentative and deny any responsibility for his or her contribution to the problem and place sole blame on the child or adolescent.
- The borderline parent may also make frequent complaints to the program staff and the supervisor about embellished and vague emotional issues.

---

[29] These are often cues or suggestions that the parent has a borderline personality.

[30] The parent may be paranoid about the patient divulging family secrets and being talked about by the patient.

[31] This is a subtle form of drama among the patient, the parent, and the clinician. The parent may try to get out of paying the copay or account balance. This seems to be in agreement with Friedman's (1989) observation that borderline personalities often try to get out of paying a bill (pp. 145–161).

The borderline parent will tend to undermine family work, and required sessions can be futile if not counterproductive.

A different set of problems occurs when the child/adolescent and parent both demonstrate borderline personalities. The patient and parent in this case are often chaotically enmeshed and mutually anxious and the parent will enable the patient to avoid treatment.[32] The parent may frequently act as the patient's spokesperson. Conversely, the parent and patient can be domestically violent toward each other. The patient and parent may attempt to draw the clinician and staff into drama with an invitation to rescue them.

Whether it is the parent or the patient, working with a borderline personality poses multiple challenges. The individual patient with borderline personality may be uncooperative and disruptive in the individual, group, and milieu settings. The borderline parent tends to deny responsibility for the child or adolescent patient's problems and is unlikely to entertain making changes to resolve family issues. Having an appreciation of these challenges is an important starting point for developing a game to work as successfully as possible with the borderline personality patient or parent.

THE GAME OF WORKING WITH
THE BORDERLINE PERSONALITY

This section suggests a game of working with the borderline personality in the PHP/IOP setting. It discusses suggested strategic paradigms and the limits of the strategies.

As elucidated in the previous section, borderline personality disorder tends to be a formidable if not gargantuan challenge. The borderline personality patient is unlikely to resolve all identified problems. Therefore when conceptualizing a game of working with a borderline personality in the PHP/IOP setting, it is more practical to identify success in terms of reasonable expectations. Success for a clinician and clinical staff in working with the patient with borderline personality disorder could include the following:

- The borderline patient does not commit suicide.
- The borderline (parent or patient) will demonstrate compliance with the treatment schedule and program format.

---

[32] This can seem insurmountable when the child/adolescent has school-refusal issues.

- The borderline patient will be discharged successfully at the end of the precertified days of treatment with a referral to an outpatient provider.
- No other patients will leave the program due to the borderline patient's behavior.
- The therapist will not be "fired" by the patient or parent for any valid reason for the duration of the patient's stay in the PHP/IOP.
- There will have been no risk management investigations of the clinician in connection with the borderline patient or parent.

In light of all of the challenges of working with a borderline personality, reasonable expectations tend to be in neutral and maybe negative terms.

The game of dealing with the borderline patient is highly abstract in the form of paradigms and activities that are not concrete. A paradigm is a conceptual framework that includes both interpretation and the set of clinician responses. By operating out of the paradigms and not a specific set of strategies, the clinician is able to appraise and understand a situation with a borderline patient from a broader base. Furthermore, a paradigm allows a clinician to develop an authentically personal style versus trying to become someone else.

The suggested game of dealing with the borderline patient consists of integrating the following core paradigms:

- Focus should be on structure and not control
- Inherent boundaries and limits should be hardwired
- Be gentle but firm
- Less is more
- This is not personal and there is nothing to prove

The paradigms can integrate or overlap in situations, but as long as the outcome is clinically appropriate, the specific paradigm being subscribed to is a peripheral matter. Some of the paradigms are redundant from Chapter 2 on the milieu and Chapter 4 on concurrent treatment planning, but the application is specific in the case of working with the patient with borderline personality disorder.

Structure and Not Control

As discussed earlier, the borderline patient's main aim in any situation is control. The borderline personality seeks to control in any situation perceived to be necessary. The borderline patient may want to choose the group and clinician. In interpersonal terms, the patient with borderline personality disorder may complain to other staff or the supervisor about the clinician in vague emotional terms. This patient's desire to control inherently conflicts with the program order and the treatment needs of other patients.

Many clinicians and staff members seek to get the borderline patient to comply with authority and end up in a dramatic and disruptive power struggle. By getting into a power struggle with the borderline personality-disordered patient, the clinician has surrendered emotional power. This patient will likely then pull the clinician into emotional drama with other staff or patients in which the clinician is portrayed as a villain or perpetrator looking unprofessional and possibly immature.

However, the paradigm of structure and control seeks to avoid the drama and conflicts by letting the borderline patient have the choice (or maybe the appearance of choice) as long as the rights and treatment of other patients are not compromised. To minimize a power and control struggle with the patient, the confrontation should be stated in terms of the program or organizational structure and not in terms of the clinician's or staff's personal control.

Inherently, this paradigm assumes a greater structure that the clinician merely represents and is required to follow. Whether parent or patient, the borderline patient should be afforded the choice when appropriate within the larger structure of the program. If the drama of a power struggle is avoided and the milieu stays calmer, then the program staff is managing the borderline patient and the milieu simultaneously. However, failing to adhere to the larger order will have consequences for the borderline personality patient, regardless of any attempt to blame the clinician. If called to give an account about a borderline patient's complaint about consequences, the clinician should be able to articulate a defense of subscribing to structure and order.[33]

Inherent Boundaries and Limits Should Be Hardwired

In addition to the borderline patient's need to control, borderline personalities tend to view clinicians and programs in both idealistic and concrete

---

[33] In this situation, the clinician emphasizes the need to follow the rules. This takes away the victim card from the borderline personality who is trying to incite drama.

terms. These views are manifested as idealistic treatment goals and idealization of clinicians and therapists. However, the borderline patient has a tendency to eventually move from idealization to rejection and repudiation of the clinician and program as a way of evading the fear of abandonment.

Many clinicians unintentionally encourage this experience of extremes when promising "to be there always" for the patient or the parent. Many patients with borderline personality disorder will test this promise by pushing, testing, and playing games with the clinician. Some of this testing includes:

- Inappropriate requests and provocative information such as disclosure about sexual peccadilloes or risky behavior
- Telling catastrophic tales about abuse or suffering
- Engaging in verbal self-abuse or deprecation while waiting for the clinician to empathize, to agree, or to rescue[34]
- Demanding special privileges such as extra individual time or permission to miss treatment for invalid reasons

Eventually, the clinician being tested will have to set limits by either confronting the patient about the behavior or saying no to a request.

After a series of tests during which the clinician must eventually say no, the borderline patient may incite drama as an angry victim. This can include criticism of the clinician as being incompetent and having abandoned the patient. The borderline patient's tendency to have a fragile ego, as translated by all-or-nothing thinking and a focus on abandonment, is a likely precipitant of the drama.

Related to the paradigm of order and control, the paradigm of hardwiring limits and boundaries inherently aims to prevent the aforementioned drama by modulating the borderline patient's idealization with subsequent limit testing. Some examples of these boundaries are seen in the following scripts:

- I'll help you as much as I can.
- I'll be here as much as I can for you.
- I will tell you if I know.

---

[34] It is not a good idea to agree with patients with borderline personality disorder when they give themselves a derogatory label. The patient may claim that the clinician gave him or her that same name or label. It may be better to avoid that and empathetically reflect that the patient is engaging in self-deprecation.

- To be honest with you, I don't think the program will help you fix everything, but it can help prepare you to get back to a point where you can _____.
- I cannot be sure, but I am confident that _____.

With this paradigm, the clinician expresses preemptive boundaries in practice.

If the borderline patient wants to press the point when a clinician tells the patient "No," the clinician has the corresponding follow-up options:

- As I have told you, I will help you as much as I can (be here for you as much as I can), and that is something I am unable to do.
- As I have said, I will tell you if I know, and in this case, I honestly do not know.
- That is one of the limits of this program.
- As I said, I was not sure.

There is no guarantee that the borderline patient will not instigate drama or make a suicidal gesture as an expression of anger in response to a clinician imposing a direct boundary after having imposed the softer boundaries. However, when the clinician thinks and acts in terms of the paradigms, he or she is better able to integrate some of the other paradigms to minimize the borderline patient's negative externalities in the milieu.

In the PHP/IOP situations in which it is the parent who has the borderline personality, the application of the hardwired boundary paradigm essentially maintains the tension. The clinician sets a boundary that is noncommittal and deferential when a parent pushes for the clinician to rescue the parent in the form of finding an impossible solution.[35] After the parental statement of the problems, some scripts the clinician can use to respond at admission include the following:

- It seems that we need to explore the problems further and see whether we are able to help.

---

[35] As noted earlier, the borderline parent typically comes in and says that none of the previous episodes of therapy have helped. There is the likelihood that the parent will disqualify most suggestions that the PHP/IOP clinician will make. The clinician is too busy with other cases to become overly invested in a creative pursuit of interventions for a borderline parent. The clinician cannot work harder than the parent.

- There are limits as to what our program is designed to do. Our program is about stabilization. I think that we may need to review what your future options are.

Tolerating tension may be a professional development matter for the clinician seeking to hardwire boundaries. The discomfort can be ameliorated with the mindfully practiced cognition that a parent must be the one to own the family problems that are occurring outside of the program; there are limits as to what the clinician can do. The parent will take ownership or will fail to take ownership of the family problem. The toleration of tension should become easier as the clinician gains experience.

In successive parent sessions, the clinician may have to maintain the tension with an exploration stance. This means the clinician spends time asking historical questions about what previous clinicians have suggested and seeking the parent's thoughts on why interventions did not work.[36] It may behoove the clinician to keep sessions involving only the parent brief and quickly move to family sessions that include the patient.[37]

Gentle but Firm

The borderline patient can be an enigma who is treatment savvy but lacks character or ego strength. When the borderline patient fails to follow through with the treatment plan goals agreed on the previous week, the clinician is existentially involved in a potentially frustrating power struggle with the patient. When the patient is either noncompliant or not invested, the clinician may be tempted to confront him or her in a strong manner, which a borderline patient cannot tolerate.

The patient with borderline personality disorder also tends to be unable to cope with confrontation delivered in a normal tone of voice. Out

---

[36] The clinician typically has to go slower than might be expected in brief therapy. However, when the particular managed care organization (MCO) gives a limit of 3 to 10 days, the clinician may have to emphasize stabilization over problem resolution and discuss what an appropriate referral should be for the patient.

[37] Often, the parent may dodge historical questions by claiming not to remember. The clinician should avoid "catching" or trapping the parent in the session but report this to the MD and in the medical record.

of an ego deficit, a borderline patient may claim that the clinician's confrontation is abrupt or allege that the clinician is yelling.[38] The borderline patient may respond in a passive-aggressive manner suggesting that the clinician is tying the patient's hands, and he or she will continue to be noncompliant with treatment. The borderline patient may claim victimhood and will demand a new clinician. As a passive-aggressive response to the confrontation, the borderline patient may drop out of treatment or engage in a passive-aggressive and possibly suicidal gesture to punish the clinician. Through these self-righteous and self-sabotaging behaviors, a borderline patient demonstrates the inability to tolerate strong confrontation and through the instigation of a subtle form of drama, claims or implicates victimization by a clinician.[39]

In the gentle-but-firm paradigm, the clinician seeks to circumvent the aforementioned cycle of behavior.[40] In this paradigm, the clinician talks to the borderline in a quiet and gentle tone about the choices that the patient is making. The clinician's word choice avoids promises or threats. The gentle-but-firm approach is a complement to the paradigm of *structure and not control*, which seeks to frame the borderline's noncompliance in the larger structural consequences, which the clinician does not control. The clinician is gently but firmly expressing that the consequences are beyond the control of the clinician, and the choices are in the patient's hands to do what is needed in treatment.[41]

The gentle-but-firm paradigm can also be applicable in the family therapy aspect of the child/adolescent PHP/IOP when dealing with the borderline parent who says that nothing works. When the clinician strongly reflects on what the parent is doing or could do differently, the parent may complain to a supervisor that the clinician is patronizing. The parent claiming patronization by the clinician will likely disrupt

---

[38] This type of embellishment suggests that some borderline patients have almost a feature off the autistic spectrum: being unable to tolerate emotion and increased volume from other individuals. If this is not autistic, it is childlike in flavor.

[39] Or the borderline patient claims that the clinician is a perpetrator.

[40] This could be called a soft skill, but it is broader than just one skill.

[41] The clinician is joining the patient in a helpless state to reduce the likelihood of tension.

treatment even if the patient was benefiting from it.[42] The clinician who is gentle and firm in conjunction with setting hardwired limits may not have productive family sessions, but he or she will reduce the likelihood of parental disruption of treatment before it has been determined that the patient's treatment benefit has been maximized.

Less Is More

Along with the gentle-but-firm paradigm comes a *less-is-more* paradigm. The more the clinician says in conversation with borderline personalities, the greater the likelihood that the borderline patient will instigate drama. Drama in these occasions includes the borderline patient embellishing the clinician's statements to staff and clinicians. Therefore, the clinician should strive to use an economy of words.

A personality disorder, including narcissistic, borderline, and antisocial personality, may tend to act confused when the clinician discusses the patient's noncompliance or defocusing behavior. Confusion can be a manifestation of the victim role and a mechanism for control. The less-is-more paradigm is informed by the structure-not-control paradigm. When the patient acts confused in what seems to be a simple situation, the clinician can exercise the less-is-more paradigm by joining with the borderline patient's confusion by saying "I'm not sure what to do here for you."[43]

It Is Not Personal, and There Is Nothing to Prove

Anger is a significant theme in working with patients with borderline personality disorder. Some newly admitted borderline patients are openly angry, critical, and intimidating, and feel entitled. As noted earlier, some borderline patients present as worried that others are angry with them. They will project anger on others. Some borderline patients will confront

---

[42] Attending to the adolescent patient's needs is complicated. It may be enough to empathize with the patient as to the difficulty of his or her situation. The discussion will gravitate eventually to the borderline parent, as the problem is of the patient getting along with the parent. The clinician should avoid direct criticism of the parent, and explore how the patient can develop coping or healthier survival skills.

[43] In this context, the clinician's move to confusion and helplessness skirts the patient's attempt to start drama.

the clinician, asking whether the clinician is angry with him or her. Some will repeat that they *just feel* the clinician is mad at them. Occasionally, an enraged borderline patient will ironically attack the clinician and claim that the clinician is angry, has anger management problems, and is in denial about them. In all of these situations, the borderline patient manifests a state of anger and assumes, perhaps obsessively, that others are reciprocating the anger.

Out of this obsession, a borderline patient tends to ask the surrounding people, including the clinician, whether they are angry with the patient. Within the less-is-more paradigm, the clinician should answer authentically, which should hopefully be "No," after which the clinician should consider setting soft limits and moving on to other tasks.

If the borderline persists in questioning whether the clinician is angry with the patient, the clinician can put the issue back to the patient. Some examples of this are the following:

- Are you judging yourself about your behavior?
- Are you feeling that I should be angry with something you just did?
- Are you feeling guilty about something right now?
- It must be tough worrying about whether people are angry with you.

There is a likelihood that the borderline patient will answer with an "I don't know" to options 1 to 3. Option 4 is a follow-up to the "I don't know." Because this does put the onus of the anger issue back on the patient, the clinician should use a firm yet gentle voice and set gentle limits with the borderline patient that include making the conversation brief.

A borderline patient may harass the clinician by persisting to insist that the clinician is angry as an attempt to gain control. The borderline patient may also instigate drama by telling other patients, the staff, and the clinician's supervisor that the clinician is angry with the patient. This patient may then embellish the clinician's statements to claim that the clinician indeed has anger management problems. In this case, the patient is claiming victimhood by creating a straw man perpetrator in the clinician.[44]

This can be a difficult situation to manage in and of itself, but the paradigm of *it is not personal and there is nothing to prove* includes the clinician's maintenance of an objective and detached view of the

---

[44] The borderline patient is the perpetrator, but is acting like both the victim and rescuer. This drama can feel as if it is perpetual, but typically lasts only a few days.

borderline patient's focus and obsession with the anger of others.[45] The borderline patient is likely defocusing from his or her issues because of the lack of ego strength and is attempting to cross emotional boundaries through accusing the clinician of being angry. The clinician can maintain objectivity by focusing on this in staffing with the psychiatrist and with the treatment team and stating the view that the patient appears to be defocusing.

This section described five paradigms that form the game of working with borderline personality-disordered patients. It is important to emphasize structure and not control remembering that the inherent boundaries are hardwired into the clinician's communication with the patient. The clinician's communication needs to be gentle but firm and use an economy of words. In the end, there is nothing to prove to the patient as the relationship is professional and not personal, and the clinician's boundaries with the patient should reflect this. These five paradigms form the basis of a professional philosophy and attitude by which a clinician can manage interactions with a borderline personality to increase the likelihood of accomplishing successful discharge from the program. The most transcendent paradigm, which these five other paradigms rest on, is that the clinician has insight and seeks to make principled and rational choices whatever the situation may be.

Limitations of the Paradigms

The paradigms will not work in all situations, but they remind us that when dealing with a borderline, the rules are different. These paradigms assume that the clinician will be allowed the time and opportunity to join with the borderline patient or parent before any crises occur. The child or adolescent with borderline personality disorder is not an adult and may need to be redirected versus being afforded negotiation. The borderline patient may also be too dysfunctional to be capable of functioning in a PHP/IOP group and milieu. Furthermore, the borderline parent has the power position in treatment in the first place and, regardless of the clinician's best work, can avoid participation or pull the child out of

---

[45] The clinician may need to be mindful that he or she is dealing with a borderline personality and that this is borderline behavior. A common borderline mantra is "It's all about me."

treatment.[46] The clinician should appreciate the limitations when interacting with a patient or parent appraised to have borderline personality traits.

The occasional case of the raging borderline patient on admission creates an awkward situation during which the clinician may have to depart from the paradigms to maintain order in the group. Sometimes this patient is guarded, defensive, and mute as part of a simple agenda to get a prescription from the psychiatrist and leave.[47] Sometimes this patient stays long enough to manifest immaturity, poor impulse control, and poor boundaries, having no respect or regard for the other PHP/IOP patients. If the newly admitted raging borderline patient causes a scene that includes inappropriate language, posturing, and verbal aggression to the other patients, the clinician may have to set firm limits and ask the patient to leave the group therapy session.[48] The raging patient who makes a scene on the day of admission in a PHP/IOP usually never returns for treatment.[49]

The adolescent with borderline traits may try to take an adult role by being critical and judgmental of other adult staff or clinicians.[50] The patient may claim victimhood because other staff or clinicians were unfair or uncaring. The patient may have to be reminded in a blunt fashion that he or she is not in charge and has to follow rules and respect authority figures.

---

[46] The reasons a borderline parent may pull a child or adolescent out prematurely include that the parent has a raging borderline personality disorder, the parent feels that the clinician is getting too close, or the parent has an undisclosed agenda that is all about himself or herself.

[47] This is more likely to occur in adult cohorts.

[48] The clinician may have to be parental in approach by making a statement such as "I'm sorry; I cannot have you act that way in this group." If the nurse's station is close by the group room door, the clinician should call another staff member to take the patient out and talk to the patient to see whether the issue can be addressed.

[49] Some patients with raging borderline personality disorder will not stay in the group but will complain to another staff member about the clinician and make the clinician a scapegoat for the patient's not wanting to stay in group therapy.

[50] By being critical and judgmental, an adolescent with borderline traits may assume an adult role with a parent with low self-esteem.

The hostile adult accusing the clinician of being angry is essentially attempting to bully the clinician emotionally to control the situation. Any such soft deflection by the clinician may result in the patient escalating the situation further and calling the clinician a liar who is in denial.[51] At this point, there is no possibility that there is a therapeutic alliance and the clinician should end the conversation and refer the patient to another clinician or discharge the patient.

This chapter has minimally touched on suicidal ideation and borderline personality, but this may be another situation that departs from the paradigms. The borderline patient who is reporting suicidal ideation and is refusing to contract for safety may either be manipulative or have a specific plan with intent. In the interest of order and safety, firm limits may need to be set in the form of placing a borderline patient on a 72-hour hold at the risk of losing the therapeutic alliance.

The borderline parent of a patient must at least communicate with the clinician for the clinician to be able to use the paradigms. A parent can dictate treatment by avoiding it. The parent may avoid clinician phone calls and then claim victimhood when the patient is discharged due to treatment noncompliance. The clinician may have to be firm when indicating that the patient is being discharged from the PHP/IOP setting because the parent did not comply with treatment as evidenced by not attending family sessions.

CONCLUSIONS

This chapter discussed working with the borderline personality in the PHP/IOP setting. It analyzed the challenges of dealing with the borderline individual and suggested a pragmatic game consisting of strategies in the form of paradigms versus following concrete behavioral steps.

This chapter was not about therapy with the borderline patient and distinctly avoided subscription to any one therapeutic school of thought. It is assumed that a typical PHP/IOP has a specific design, plan, and schedule, and the borderline patient is going to comply

---

[51] This patient is trying to reverse patient and clinician roles through intimidation.

within that structure or will not stay in treatment. The treatment will likely be short term, and the patient may reap limited benefit from the program design. The suggested strategies in this chapter tend to enhance the borderline patient's likelihood of benefitting from PHP/IOP treatment, regardless of the clinician's therapeutic approach, so that the patient can return to regular functioning while fostering a greater sense of order.

Working with the borderline parent provides different challenges. The borderline parent's child or adolescent may have been in psychiatric treatment multiple times due to parental dysfunction. The borderline parent typically wants change in the patient, but lacks insight into his or her contribution to the problem and will take no responsibility. Many parents in these cases are avoidant of family therapy sessions, which will shorten treatment. The PHP/IOP does what it can in these cases.

Although this is not a diagnostic chapter, the challenges discussed here are inherently signals that the individual patient or the parent may have a borderline personality. If the clinician realizes that one of these challenges is occurring, it is time to start playing or executing the game by mindfully applying one or more of the paradigms.

The game of working with the borderline patient in the PHP/IOP is more abstract than the other games suggested in this book, and it is up to the clinician's discretion as to how to apply the paradigms in light of the challenges. The paradigms suggested in this chapter can appear to be redundant with previous discussions despite different aims and applications.

The paradigms of the game of working with the borderline patient in the PHP/IOP setting are intended to work within the other games discussed in this book. The clinician can utilize the five paradigms during treatment planning, family therapy, and group therapy, and when addressing the social problems within the milieu. These paradigms are foundational approaches that help maintain appropriate boundaries among the patient, the clinician, and the program.

Countertransference by clinicians and staff toward borderline patients, which takes the form of natural responses of anger and dread, is normal. Indeed, the borderline patient creates headaches and turmoil for all the surrounding people, including the clinical staff. At times, the borderline patient can seem to be working on anything but treatment, and the staff members seem focused on fending off the patient's latest salvo or attack. When difficult patients with borderline personality disorder are discharged, staff members may experience a brief feeling of relief. Although countertransference is normal, it is hoped that over time, the clinician and staff can shift paradigms from natural emotional reactions to a mindful attitude that includes the following:

- This is borderline personality with all of its challenges.
- This is what is required for competent treatment in our situation.
- These are the limits of what we can do for the borderline patient.
- We are professional in our approach.

REFERENCES

Friedman, W. H. (1989). *Practical group therapy: A guide for clinicians.* San Francisco, CA: Jossey-Bass.

Lenzenweger, M. F., Lane, M. C., Loranger, A. W., & Kessler, R. C. (2007). DSM-IV personality disorders in the National Comorbidity Survey Replication. *Biological Psychiatry, 62,* 553–564.

Yalom, I., & Leszcz, M. (2005). *The theory and practice of group psychotherapy* (5th ed.). New York, NY: Basic Books.

CHAPTER FIFTEEN

A DEATH IN THE PROGRAM

Given that psychiatric treatment involves humans, it is a real possibility that a clinician will experience the death of a patient during the course of a career. Some of the patients will die of natural causes, addiction issues, or by accident. Some of the patients will take their own lives.

There is significant material written about the personal issues faced by a clinician when a patient commits suicide. This body of work suggests steps to follow both to minimize liability and to include considerations for the clinician's own mental health, but there is little formally published discussion[1] about how to address a patient death in a group or milieu setting.

Patients do die in the partial hospitalization program (PHP)/intensive outpatient program (IOP) setting. There will be suicides as well as natural deaths. This chapter briefly discusses possible actions a clinician needs to take with other patients when a patient dies.

Theoretically, in terms of managing a therapeutic milieu, the principle of order suggests that patient deaths be handled in a principled manner. DiBella and colleagues (1982) suggest that if a patient does commit suicide, the matter should be made a community matter and dealt with in an open fashion.[2]

The following list offers some suggested evaluation questions to use to determine whether disclosure of a patient death to the group is necessary:

- Was the patient's death a result of natural causes or suicide?
- Was the deceased patient connected to and close to the other current patients in the program?

---

[1] One unpublished Internet article was found on dealing with a patient suicide in an inpatient unit.

[2] They also suggest when there is a significant suicide attempt by a patient, it should be discussed in the group.

- ■ Was the deceased patient enmeshed with other current patients?
- ■ Are other patients asking about the deceased patient or express-
  ing knowledge about the death?
- • What was the nature of the patient's death?
- • Was there an emotional reaction by staff members; are they affected
  in a way that will be noticeable to patients?

Overall, not all patient deaths must be disclosed and processed
with the milieu or group. Each situation should be evaluated using the
preceding questions as to the death's clinical impact on the milieu. Not
every patient will have formed bonds with the rest of the group due to
short stays in the program. There are some patient deaths that are natural
and not due to suicide. The information that the patient died may not be
discovered until several days afterward, when a significant number of
discharges have occurred. The patient population may have turned over
sufficiently so that the matter is irrelevant to the current set of patients,
and disclosure of the patient death may cause only undue distress to
acute patients.

If it is indicated that the suicide or death is to be disclosed, the clinician should make the disclosure in the group. The clinician should process the loss with the group, assess patients for safety, and make whatever
arrangements are necessary to ensure safety. The clinician should attend
to and validate patient feelings.

The clinician also has an opportunity to educate the group about
suicide, death, and grief and loss. Patients with depression and anxiety
may have a subtle break from reality and need some grounding about the
normalcy of having various negative feelings in response to loss.

If a program has more than one therapy group of the same cohort
running simultaneously and the patients of the groups interact in some
fashion before sessions, during breaks, or after program hours, the groups
could be merged for the disclosure.[3] Merging of the groups briefly for

---

[3] Depending on the caps set by Medicare and Medicaid, and on how the organization interprets the regulations, the larger group may not be billable. However,
if there is one therapist for each capped quantity (one clinician for the maximum of 10 or 12) and the clinician is billing for and documenting for that set of
patients, billing is unlikely to be a problem.

this purpose provides an opportunity to maintain continuity in how the matter is processed.

The group session in which a patient's death is announced can be conducted as follows: The designated clinician or staff member should open the group with the disclosure and then offer the group members a chance to express feelings or make statements. When patients ask questions about details, the facts should be disclosed in good taste[4] as much as possible within applicable privacy laws. When the group appears to be finished, it is appropriate to move on to patient topics for the remainder of the session.

The patients in the group may present as overly emotional in processing a patient suicide, as psychiatric acuity and rationality can present as opposites. Some anxious patients may express survivors' guilt and verbalize a fear that the PHP/IOP setting is a dangerous place and that they are unsure that they want to stay. Some patients may become suicidal and unable to contract for safety; they may need to be referred for inpatient stabilization. The clinician dealing with this situation for the first time may feel like an actor, as he or she maintains a calm and orderly demeanor for the group, even if personally shaken.[5]

If chaplaincy services are available, they can be a soothing resource in such situations. It can be helpful to have a chaplain cofacilitate the

---

[4] Staff should not volunteer facts until patients ask questions. The patient's method of suicide should not be discussed. In smaller localities, newspapers/media may report the cause of death anyway.

[5] A clinician should maintain emotional boundaries and not make an unsolicited disclosure of personal feeling unless a patient poses a direct question and avoiding answering it would cause more disruption than answering it. The clinician's answer in these occasions should be framed as a normal human reaction. An example is "Yes, it does hurt that he (or she) took his (or her) own life." Personal disclosure of such feeling does open the risk of a personality-disordered patient trying to reverse roles with a clinician. The clinician needs to set polite and firm limits with a patient who continues to ask a clinician about personal issues. An example of this plan would be a scripted response such as "I thank you for your concern, but the issues at hand are your issues and are why you need to be here in treatment."

group with the clinician(s), offer spiritual perspectives, and perhaps close the group with an ecumenical or mission-related prayer/benediction.[6]

Before or after the patients have been attended to, it is helpful for clinicians and staff to consider processing the death among themselves. It can be helpful to talk about shock and feelings resulting from the patient's death. Listening to each other's feelings is one of the important ways staff members support each other.

It is crucial for the clinician and staff to move on emotionally and behaviorally after a patient death, because the current patients are still there and have needs. It is normal for a clinician to analyze and ruminate on what could have been done differently. Clinicians also can ruminate on the fear that risk management and regulatory investigators will uncover issues that the clinician should have addressed. For the most part, the clinician has no more control over the situation, and any rumination is a distraction from the intense workload that typically sits in front of a clinician.[7]

CONCLUSIONS

This chapter offered an orderly strategy for dealing with patient deaths. Each situation must be evaluated as to whether or not disclosure should be made to the group. If disclosure about the death is made to and processed with the group, it should revolve around the feelings and safety of the group members, and the clinician should only make a personal disclosure if asked a direct question by a patient. When the patient death is shocking to the clinician and staff, it could be helpful to process this privately so as to maintain good patient–professional boundaries. Even if they are still in shock, it is critical for the clinician and staff to move on to the issues of the current patients.

---

[6] Chaplains typically have general prayers they can use to accommodate the widest range of beliefs, including "God of our understanding." If the chaplain is a Catholic priest, the connotation is generally going to be accepted that the prayer may be Catholic in nature.

[7] If an employee assistance program (EAP) is available, it may be suitable to get an appointment and process feelings in these occasions.

Patient deaths are going to happen, and they do happen in the PHP/IOP setting. They are a growth experience for all involved.

Patient deaths will still be a shock, but it is crucial for the clinical staff to be orderly and principled versus being reactive in dealing with patient deaths. Professionalism assumes that the clinician has experience and practice knowledge in handling such situations. The reality is that the inexperienced clinician must have a first experience in dealing with a patient death. Having a plan to keep a calm face and controlled demeanor in such situations is a good start.

REFERENCE

DiBella, G., Weitz, G., Poynter-Berg, D., & Yurmark, J. L. (1982). *Handbook of partial hospitalization*. New York, NY: Brunner/Mazel.

CHAPTER SIXTEEN

PROBLEMS WITH COLLEAGUES AND OTHER DEPARTMENTS

Many of us who felt that a career in the helping professions was going to be a meaningful vocation dreamed that we could help people, feel fulfilled doing it, and that was going to be it. In our quest for meaning, we eschewed the quest for wealth in favor of the pursuit of making a difference in the people's lives. We sought intrinsic value in the forms of meaning and fulfillment. Many of us did not necessarily take into account that we would have headaches caused by our coworkers. Many of us assumed that everyone we would work with in the helping professions would be genuine, cooperative, and pleasant, and we would all be successful and happy. A cruel wake-up call is that nothing is further from the truth.

Toxic work environments have been a hidden secret in the mental health and social services professions. This is not typically discussed in clinical coursework. There is no research seeking to understand the extent and causation of toxic work environments in the mental health and social services sector.[1] Where there are toxic work environments, top administration in those agencies often present as occupied with their own tasks and pursuits while distant and aloof from those at the street level.[2]

---

[1] Although there is no known data about mental health workplace hostility, research by the Centers for Disease Control and Prevention (2010) suggests a higher prevalence of hostile workplaces in the health care sector (9.1%) than in all other employment sectors combined (7.8%): http://www.cdc.gov/niosh/topics/nhis/pdfs/HealthcareOccupationProfile.pdf

[2] Brendtro and Mitchell, in their chapter in the book by Brendtro and Ness (1983), discuss the dysfunctional organization in child residential care, including the chasm between administration and the line-level worker.

As in other treatment and service settings, partial hospitalization program (PHP)/intensive outpatient program (IOP) environments can be toxic and problematic. The toxic work environment, combined with the intensity of the therapeutic milieu, can cause as much if not more stress than working with difficult patients. In many agencies, a clinician may find it easier to relate to patients than colleagues, giving credence to the joke that the only difference between staff and the patients is who has the name tags and keys. The toxic workplaces increase the probability of staff burnout and frequent turnover.

Although some professionals have a career plan that includes rapid advancement and frequent job change, others desire a stable environment and long-term employment in one place. Others have a job history that is a series of escaping one dysfunctional work environment for another in the pursuit of greener pastures. Finding that work environment where coworkers are committed and mature professionals may be equivalent to searching for that elusive pot of gold at the end of the rainbow. If a good work environment, especially in the PHP/IOP setting, is to be found, it will have to be created and maintained through the cooperation of the current occupants.

This chapter offers suggestions for the reader to negotiate toxic work environments that will lead to the creation of positive PHP/IOP work environments, given collegial problems both inside and outside of the department. This chapter discusses options for action and coping with the unchangeable.

THE CHALLENGES IN GENERAL

The reality is that all of us are human, and we will face some problems that can be resolved and some situations that are unchangeable. Some of the unchangeable problems concern helping professionals who are unhealthy individuals in and of themselves. Some of them present as having an ego lacuna in that they espouse coping skills and healthy living, but ironically appear to eschew those skills and habits in their personal lives. These unhealthy professionals exhibit anxiety, immaturity, passive-aggressiveness, abusiveness, and general incivility in coworker relationships to the point of presenting as dysfunctional, if not pathological.

Any individual in an organization can be dysfunctional. No organizational level is excluded. There can be dysfunctional psychiatrists, nurses, administrators, clinicians, and support personnel.

This dysfunction breeds toxic and hostile work environments with workplace bullying and drama that eventually affect the quality of patient care. Workplace drama can present as competitions to see who can make the other look incompetent by pointing out perceived clinical mistakes. Patients can be triangulated into employee drama, which engenders chaos and degrading of treatment focus. The chaos and perceived lack of successful treatment outcomes diminish the intrinsic value of the work as well as work satisfaction. This chaos also precipitates job burnout, which leads disillusioned, young clinicians to leave the profession despite all the time, effort, and resources they spent on education and credentialing.

It is held here that barring ethical laxness, two of the largest manifestations of pathology in the mental health or human services organization are drama and lack of emotional intelligence.[3] As discussed in Chapter 2, drama is a common problem in therapeutic milieus, but it also is a problem among staff members in an organization. In terms of an organization, drama can be:

- An unintentional occurrence arising from ignorance or impulsivity
- A lack of boundaries between employees or staff
- A habit with no other discernible cause
- Evidence that significant anger or anxiety exists among employees
- A manifestation of an individual's lack of ego strength[4]
- A deliberate act of malevolence[5]

Essentially, drama is immature and unprofessional communication.

In the cases of drama, there is a limit as to what the supervisor can do. Sometimes, complaining to a supervisor about the drama of a coworker may only perpetuate the drama, based on the supervisor's management

---

[3] There are individuals with Machiavellian and utilitarian values and standards. Out of these values and standards, they can present as perfidious and malevolent in decisions and actions if it serves their purposes. The opposite of the Machiavellian and utilitarian views would be altruism and integrity.

[4] As discussed in Chapter 2, a staff member with low emotional intelligence has a risk of getting pulled into patient drama. It is possible that this same staff member will perpetuate and escalate the drama to the point where it stops having anything to do with a patient but becomes about the staff member.

[5] Workplace bullying could take the form of drama where one form of bullying is the instigation of rumors and embellished allegations.

style, emotional intelligence, and experience level. There also may be a limit as to how much a supervisor is interested in or capable of addressing drama and poor coworker boundaries.

The matter of boundaries among staff members is a consideration in the drama. Whereas patient–staff boundaries are formal and defined, boundaries among the staff are not. The degree of worker experience, mindfulness, and intention affect the observance and respect of these coworker boundaries. Some staff members assume that the boundaries in the workplace are similar to the boundaries in their families and touch things in coworkers' workspaces and take things. Some immature coworkers cross boundaries in passive-aggressive ways by hiding various objects[6] or mocking and gossiping about each other. A clinician lacking distress tolerance can cross boundaries by meddling with another clinician's case management efforts by acting as a rescuer when hearing a patient characterize problems as catastrophic. A PHP/IOP staff member with poor interpersonal boundaries will tend to have more drama and chaos.

There is an interplay between the perpetuation of drama and a lack of emotional intelligence. A person lacking emotional intelligence and insight tends to react emotionally and impulsively when attacked in the midst of drama.[7] Or a lack of insight into drama tends to breed confusion when an assumed victim or assumed rescuer instigates drama. If drama among employees is unchecked, it can:

• Destroy morale
• Inhibit staff cooperation
• Reduce staff effectiveness
• Diminish the program reputation
• Affect the bottom line

A new or novice clinician starting work in such a toxic work environment can become consumed to the point of experiencing shaken confidence and identity. In the first 90 days, toxic coworkers with poor

[6] Examples of the passive-aggressive behavior include coffee cups being hidden, desks being rifled through, or necessary equipment subtly hidden or moved.

[7] Even with developed emotional intelligence, it seems that there is a potential for anyone to get subsumed into drama if the salient trigger is manifested. The trigger is typically an embellishment and distortion of reality. Drama tends to happen rapidly if not instantaneously.

boundaries can wield inappropriate influence in masking drama as concerns about the probationary clinician's ability to do the job. The clinician actually may be competent in doing the work, but toxic colleagues who perpetuate drama feed into splitting by patients and then voice unsupportive or unconstructive criticism in the guise of worry about the new clinician's ability. The instigation of this drama by these colleagues could present as workplace bullying and sabotage of new employees.[8]

Drama does not occur just among individuals within the PHP/IOP departments, it can occur in connection with other individuals outside the department and the organization for whatever reason. It is possible that organization employees from outside the department can instigate drama. The ones outside of the organization instigating the drama may be a referral source or bear some kind of oversight authority.

The natural outcome of the drama tends to be escalation of anger, anxiety, or distrust. The drama instigated by individuals outside of the department can present as that person:

- Crossing appropriate role boundaries (being the perpetrator)
- Acting as the reporter of embellished or emotional allegations (being the rescuer)[9]
- Complaining to one staff member about a third colleague (acting as the victim)[10]

The drama can be complicated because the individual from outside the department may have legitimacy to enter the department and interact with patients for official purposes such as payment collection or quality assurance.

FINDING ONE'S BEARINGS

Before discussing a game of dealing with some of these aforementioned coworker problems, some self-reflection is in order to find one's bearings. Much energy and focus can be diverted from clinical work to the

---

[8] This intrusion by the incumbent coworker reflects poor clinical judgment in the first place.

[9] This could be done out of ignorance or it could be done with some sense of malice.

[10] An outside instigator will likely tell an organization employee with whom he or she is familiar or has a personal relationship.

survival of the toxic behavior and drama emanating from a dysfunctional coworker or work environment. Coworker conflict can emotionally consume anyone to the point of distraction and even confusion.

Getting consumed by the coworker drama can make a clinician lose bearings. Why is the clinician there? Is it to engage in mature and competent professional clinical practice or is it to survive the drama instigated by coworkers at all costs? Hopefully, the game of handling problems with coworkers is to minimize our distraction from the important client work.

The average clinician is a highly motivated professional who has attained advanced education and who is internally motivated to get work done without the need of close supervision. Such professionals are guided by principles and logic in the manner in which they do their work. A professional should demonstrate mature composure in the workplace with both patients and coworkers. The quality of the clinician's work and conduct should be measured by professional standards and relevant codes of ethics. If the game of dealing with coworker problems is played with nothing less than integrity and principle, the clinician will present as a mere manipulator lacking character.

In contrast to the matter of character in some of the toxic workplaces, the office politics consist of staff doing nothing but playing a toxic, competitive game. Many staff members who are doyennes or doyens have refined playing a toxic, survival game because of their perceived need to survive. This toxic game includes inciting drama and passive-aggressively sabotaging other employees. Some present as having no insight as to why they have played the game.

It follows that if a professional clinician is going to play the game of dealing with staff problems in an above-board manner, he or she should be able to defend such strategies on the basis of a mature application of a principle. Challenging and toxic inquisitors may insinuate and question the clinician's motivation as being nefarious or malevolent. When playing the games of dealing with coworker problems in a toxic work environment, there can be sophisticated attacks on integrity or character that may be preposterous. The professional should be able to respond to these challenges with a calm attitude of humility, because the clinician is always abiding by and applying a principle.

In light of the pursuit of principle, a clinician may have to evaluate whether it is detrimental to stay in a position when the work environment presents as highly toxic with a majority of dysfunctional members. Some work environments are not going to improve because of the departmental and organizational status quo. There is a family system dynamic, if not an economic dynamic, in such departments in which one action of confronting a problem will result in a number of hostile reactions or externalities, including instigation of further drama. The equilibrium of such a status quo can bring about an escalation of attacks on a clinician to the point of ironic and misguided labeling as a troublemaker to the point of wrongful termination.[11] Such a chaotic work environment may be so stressful that it is causing physical harm.

THE GAME IN GENERAL

The suggested game of dealing with staff problems is similar to the milieu management strategies offered in Chapter 2, but for the purposes of this discussion, is called *drama management*. Drama management is an internalized strategy whereby a clinician first sifts information about the behavior and statements of others through three critical questions or filters of source and form:

- Is this the behavior of a mature adult or is it immature emotion?
- Is this drama or a subdued reporting of fact?
- What (if anything) is needed?

After determining whether it is fact or drama, the next phase of the game is an application of passive or active boundaries. The third phase of the game requires one take a leadership role in the active creation of a positive work environment. This section elaborates on the strategy and its application.

Mature Adult Behavior Versus Immature Emotion

The first filter determines the emotional stance of the coworker. A sufficient theoretical base to borrow from is *transactional analysis* (Berne, 1964/2004) with its suggested structure of *parent, adult,* and *child* ego or

---

[11] When describing the dysfunctional coworker to an outside party or authority, the reporter may feel that he or she is sounding equally dysfunctional.

emotional states. The parent state uses a didactic tone of communicating to another person as one would to a child.[12] The adult state uses the mature stance with which a person demonstrates self-control, emotional regulation, and calmness. The adult acting in the child state demonstrates:

- Immature angry or intolerant behavior
- Dwelling on worry
- Impulsive reactivity to situations

The significance of the filter is that the immature adult focused on emotion demonstrates poor judgment and is not credible.

Is This Drama or a Subdued Report of Fact?

Another aspect of this strategy is filtering whether the information is a rational and logical report of facts or drama. The three subcomponents of this filtering component include the following critical questions:

- Is the information actual fact or merely emotion?
- Who is the actual channel of the information?
- Is there a need for action?

Emotional communication in drama is about the feelings and not the fact. It is focused around how something was said or received versus what was actually said.[13] There may be a modicum of truth, but it is not accurately represented. The subject matter is often judgmental criticism in general terms but lacks specificity. If the subject matter is specific, it involves an allegation that is emotionally laden and sensational. As discussed elsewhere in the book, drama also tends to offer a distorted characterization of emotion or an embellishment of a situation.

An instigation or perpetuation of drama tends to present in three general forms:

---

[12] The parental tone varies as to situation, but the receiver of the message often feels patronized.

[13] Examples of emotional communication are "He was pushy." "You do not have to be abrupt about it." "He talked down to me like I was a little child."

- The person claims to be a victim of emotional harm.
- The rescuer educates a victim.[14]
- The rescuer confronts an identified perpetrator.[15]

The channel through which the subject matter comes also can suggest whether or not it is an instigation of drama. One such channel is a side party claiming to represent the complaint of one or more people. Another such channel is a third party relating the information after the fact.[16] It is likely that information that is not directly reported through established complaint channels for filing complaints is an instigation of drama.

Drama has been called passive-aggressive communication in that, on the one hand, the person acts passively and on the other, acts aggressively. The opposite of drama is the offended party showing the character strength to either ignore a petty offense or assertively confront the offending party about the problem in a straightforward manner.

The significance of this filter is to evaluate the validity and reliability of the "concern." In the process of the evaluation, the clinician can practice some emotional regulation versus jumping to conclusions that there is a true problem or complaint.

What Is Needed?

A third strategy of this game is evaluating what is needed. When dysfunctional coworkers are dwelling on worries or complaining about the extraneous, there is no specific and realistic solution to the problem. However, individuals acting in a dysfunctional manner present worries and resentments as concrete problems. These worries are also unsolvable, yet they are looking for a solution. If the individual dwelling on a problem

---

[14] Examples of this are "He wants to fight you." "Do you know what she said about you?" "Do you know what she did?"

[15] Examples can include "What did you do to that person?" "Why did you do that?"

[16] In some patient situations, this information should be acted on in cases in which one patient relates the threats of another patient's threats of physical harm to a fourth party.

responds to the question of "What is needed?" with "I don't know," then it appears that the coworker does not have a real problem.

On the other hand, when the solution requires an absent third party to make a choice, then the individual is engaging in worry. Worry is a form of anxiety in which an individual is focused on matters that are out of his or her control or that cannot be solved at that time. There typically is no realistic action that can solve another person's worry.

The Application of Boundaries

In some ways, drama is like energy and the responses to it will either intensify and perpetuate it or keep it from advancing by absorption. An emotional reaction to drama tends to complete a triangle of communication through engendering a further act of rescue, claim of victimhood, or perceived perpetration. An insightful response or reaction recognizes the instigation or perpetuation of drama and applies a boundary that theoretically inhibits completion of a triangular pattern of communication. Some of these responses or reactions include:

- Being direct and confronting coworkers without intermediaries
- Not repeating an instigating comment to another person
- Requesting that the third party (colleague or patient) come and talk directly
- Refusing to rescue someone portraying himself or herself as a victim
- Not discussing a matter when confronted by the third party
- Offering an apology to the third party when the confrontation seems perfidious
- Ignoring

Although there is a likelihood of precipitating reactionary drama, direct and assertive confrontation of an offending coworker when necessary is a priority in demonstrating character and professionalism. If the coworker presents as significantly toxic, a soft and firm tone of voice may neutralize the complaint that the clinician was abrupt. Eye contact and good posture are essential nonverbal communication tools that compensate for a soft tone. One has greater power when confronting a coworker in private versus with an audience, because there are fewer individuals to embellish what happened. If the offending coworker has recruited rescuers to confront the clinician for alleged perpetration, the clinician should set another boundary by politely refusing to discuss or repeat the matter.[17]

The boundary of not repeating an instigating comment can be a mere act of ignoring the matter or a strategic control move. Assuming that a dysfunctional person's instigation of drama is gossip in the form of relating another person's anger or complaint about still another person in emotional terms, not repeating it minimizes the profile and power of the instigator.

The person instigating drama by claiming victimhood may be tempting to assist. However, if the alleged offense is evaluated to be drama, agreeing to mediate or intercede is likely going to thrust the rescuer into the drama. The appropriate boundary in this case is empathy with a statement of regret of an inability to help, and that the matter is between the alleged victim and alleged perpetrator.[18]

A firm, if not aggressive, boundary to set when being confronted by a peer for an alleged offense by another peer is a refusal to discuss the matter. Typically, the tone needs to be gentle but firm. The volume used should be between a normal speaking voice and almost a whisper. The language in such a case should be a terse and assertive, "I am not going to discuss this with you. This is between me and her/him." The flip side is to tell a "rescuer" to have the person come to you directly. In the case of patient–staff splitting, a boundary is to tell a colleague or coworker to refer a patient back to the clinician.[19] To maintain this boundary, it may

---

[17] The script to say to the rescuers is "This is between me and him (or her)." If the supervisor gets involved, the clinician should indeed discuss the matter and how it was explored in a professional and ethical manner.

[18] Sometimes, the drama may be an invitation to engage in cooperating in making a formal complaint against a supervisor.

[19] Telling a coworker to send patients back to the clinician is a test of the coworker's dysfunction. Many coworkers will comply with the request without incident. A coworker who refuses to comply with the request or who supports the patient's emotional complaint reveals much about his or her dysfunction.

be necessary to sound repetitive, like a broken record, in the refusal to discuss the matter.[20, 21]

One other option for managing drama is not necessarily setting a boundary, but is going immediately and offering a humble apology just in case there is some validity to the confrontation that one offended a third party. This is an assertive and strategic move made to preserve a relationship when it appears a rescuer is trying to split or create discord between the receiver and an alleged victim. In this case, the information is evidenced to be a perfidious portrayal of a third person's emotional distress. One has confirmation that this was drama when the alleged victim either presents as confused or denies that there ever was a problem.

An appropriate follow-up for processing the confusion is openly identifying what happened as an attempt to instigate drama or split staff. This follow-up properly strengthens healthy relationships and can appropriately marginalize the instigator. A subtle part of drama management is educating healthier peers about the instigation of drama. Such a discussion should be conducted in a humble and calm tone. The lower tone and emotional level demonstrate character and are crucial for lessening the likelihood that any further drama will be engendered by the matter.[22]

---

[20] To sound like a broken record, one should go slower and softer, not louder and faster. If the coworker persists after a few repetitions, it may be necessary to get up and leave and report this inappropriate behavior on the coworker's part, which is creating a hostile workplace, to the supervisor or to corporate compliance (where applicable). When contemplating making the report to the supervisor or corporate compliance, it seems more mature to abstain from making a threat and to act without warning. The act of making a threat has a potential inflammatory effect.

[21] If the supervisor is the one doing the confronting, then the supervisor is entitled to a factual discussion of what happened or what the alleged perpetrator thinks happened. A typical scenario in these cases is that the alleged victim is mad that the alleged perpetrator either set an earlier limit or declined to perform a favor. However, if the supervisor is shown to be an actual instigator of the drama, it may constitute workplace bullying and thus necessitate reporting through appropriate channels. Such a report about a supervisor will need to be substantiated in the form of a paper trail or at least one to two other individuals who can corroborate the information.

[22] Being able to process the drama in this manner may increase one's informal power level, stature, or influence in a department.

One last suggested boundary involves the passive act of ignoring a dysfunctional colleague's noisiness. Many dysfunctional individuals are verbose in their chronic, anxious complaining or angry tirades, which tend to be self-focused. This is intentional ignoring, informed by the perspective that the chronic complaining is immature and unprofessional behavior on the colleague's part. The colleague's immature behavior has the potential to precipitate drama if another individual tries to confront, rescue, or soothe the emotional colleague. Although some minimal empathy of the colleague's pain is in order, ignoring reduces the probability of being pulled into the drama that could emanate from the negative colleague's chronic complaining.

This section discussed the game of drama management. It is a reactive game that looks at the larger picture of what is happening. The strategies suggested are about evaluating the form, tone, and pathways of the information and then reacting in ways that lessen the likelihood that drama is perpetuated. One can react through inactive and active boundaries. Drama tends to happen quickly, because emotion engenders impulsivity. When there is a toxic environment, the game of drama management requires the clinician to practice a slowing down reaction while seeking to increase the use of critical thinking skills in interactions with coworkers.

Leading in the Creation of a Positive Work Environment

The bulk of this chapter has been about strategically reacting to the negative dynamics of dysfunctional individuals and managing interactions. An important simultaneous strategy to use when responding to the negative is leadership in the creation of a positive work environment. Like the discussion of the therapeutic milieu earlier, the work environment is also a type of economy in that there can be positive and negative externalities based on the inputs.

Also like the therapeutic milieu, a good work environment is not entirely created by accident. Merely reacting in a healthy manner to toxic behavior does not make for a positive environment. Although there are frustrating physical settings and leadership decisions that negatively affect the environment,[23] the clinician and colleagues can proactively

---

[23] Physical space issues can include temperature, space, and mold. Leadership may make decisions without evaluation or consultation of line-level staff who are ignorant of crucial issues.

improve its quality and comfortableness through attitudes, generosity, and demonstration of character.

Attitude

For the purpose of this discussion, *attitude* is the combination of what one thinks and how one feels. The most important attitude that a clinician can have is a *can do* attitude versus an *I don't know if I can do it* attitude. The clinician is a professional and is paid to do difficult things. Difficult things are not impossible things. The *can do* attitude is balanced by an attitude of *humility*, as no one is perfect and sometimes everyone needs assistance in accomplishing a quantity of work or tackling a problematic situation.[24] The professional who has appropriate humility asks for assistance from team members or colleagues when necessary.

Be Generous to Your Coworkers Within Appropriate Boundaries and Means

Part of a healthy work environment is generosity among individuals, which can come in many forms. A clinician can be generous in the form of affirmations by complimenting colleagues on their good work and telling them that it is good to work with them. It can come in the form of helping colleagues complete other tasks when they are dealing with a crisis without an expectation of a return favor. A popular form of generosity is bringing food for coworkers and celebrating events such as birthdays. Generosity in all of its forms is an investment in the office atmosphere.

If there has been a history of toxicity in a workplace, the practice of generosity may be received with awkwardness and suspicion. Colleagues accustomed to being on guard and reactive may exhibit confusion and anxiety in response to initial acts of generosity. The motivation of a generous clinician also may be considered suspect. Practicing and promoting generosity in a work environment may be an educational process. Furthermore, generosity without character otherwise presents as manipulation.

---

[24] A case may be confusing for the clinician or the clinician may have some doubts about how to handle a situation.

Character

Character, for the purposes of this discussion, includes the practice of integrity and ethical values. It includes abstaining from gossip or criticism of coworkers behind their backs. It also includes confronting a coworker directly when appropriate or reporting inappropriate behavior to the management in a factual matter and not repeating it to other coworkers. A clinician with character will stand up for what is honest and ethically right but will also respect different theoretical schools of thought. Character includes treating all coworkers with dignity and respect. Finally, character should be a motivation for apologizing when a clinician is wrong or incorrect. Character builds a foundation of trust among coworkers and is a sign of professional maturity.

This section discussed the strategy of leading in the creation of a positive work environment. A positive work environment is more likely to exist when the workers demonstrate a positive attitude toward work. Generosity in both tangible and intangible forms is also an investment toward engendering belonging and acceptance in the workplace. Finally, creating such a work environment requires character. If these leadership strategies do not reform the workplace environment, they at least add intrinsic value when there are unchangeable toxic externalities that make a workplace difficult.

COPING WITH THE UNCHANGEABLE

Toxic or dysfunctional workplaces exist and can present as unchangeable,[25] and those with longevity in those settings either tend to be on that same level of dysfunction or have resolved to cope and tolerate it. Coping and tolerating are commitments.

---

[25] This chapter does not suggest why workplaces remain toxic. There is no research on this for mental health settings. It seems that if appropriate existing datasets were to be identified, factor analysis or ordinary least-squares regression analysis could inexpensively suggest insights into the toxicity. Otherwise, workplace toxicity or dysfunction could be a topic for a quantitative dissertation if a grant could be secured. A study that seeks to measure the economic value of lost productivity due to drama among coworkers in mental health settings would also be interesting research that could motivate further research and change.

The reaction to workplace toxicity may have some similarity to Kübler-Ross's (1969) five-stage grief process of denial, anger, bargaining, depression, and acceptance. The revelation of toxicity is a form of loss, and clinicians may struggle through anger at themselves and others. In addition to the anger resulting from the abuse, there may be feelings of guilt[26] about the work problems. The clinician may bargain internally and externally regarding whether there are things that can be done to remain in the position.[27] The clinician may then feel depressed when it is evident that there is no more bargaining that can be done. The clinician is engaging in an emotional process with both professional and personal aspects.

The newly hired clinician who is working through the consuming emotions resulting from workplace toxicity has both a difficult learning curve and must engage in a decision-making process as to whether staying in the job is worth the stress and strain. In some ways, the decision to leave is easier if the clinician feels that an extended probation or other employee discipline measure based on colleague input is unfair. The clinician may continue to engage in bargaining by staying in the job despite feeling little loyalty to the supervisor and organization. In the end, it may prove necessary for one's emotional and physical health to leave a toxic workplace.

The longer a clinician stays in an organization, the more unchangeable workplaces become manifest. The clinician shows acceptance of the situation by tolerance or avoidance when possible. Life's other priorities, such as providing for a spouse and family, engender an existential resolve in the clinician to move a dysfunctional workplace from the center of focus by compartmentalization and concentration on personal matters. Achieving this life–work balance enables a clinician to cope and still do meaningful work despite a dysfunctional workplace with toxic coworkers.

CONCLUSIONS

This chapter discussed negotiation of toxic work situations and how to lead as a change agent in the creation of positive PHP/IOP work

---

[26] Guilt in this case is the clinician's self-directed anger. The clinician may feel guilt for not recognizing the dysfunction in the workplace before accepting the job.

[27] Part of this bargaining may be getting involved in the drama and arguments with coworkers who are crossing boundaries versus actually setting boundaries.

environments. It reviewed the challenges of workplace toxicity and options for action and coping with the unchangeable.

Workplace drama is a significant dysfunction or toxicity that occurs throughout mental health and social service workplaces including PHP/IOP settings. It is an element of hostile work environments that has multiple causes. It can take the form of workplace bullying. Nuisance drama also occurs with individuals from outside of the department. Drama is an immature communication pattern that is symptomatic of poor emotional intelligence, poor clinical judgment, and poor social judgment. It engenders higher employee turnover and the delivery of inferior clinical services.

The game of dealing with toxic coworkers and transforming the work environment has two strategic components: drama management and leadership in a positive work environment. Drama management is a reactionary strategy that combines critically evaluating communication according to its source and form with responding in calculated ways that lessen the likelihood that drama is perpetuated. The other half of the game consists of a proactive strategy of leading in the development of a positive workplace through use of a positive attitude, generosity, and the demonstration of character. This game of dealing with drama can be difficult, if not taxing.

Recognizing drama, and responding to it in strategic or tactical ways, requires a moral compass in which the clinician has found his or her bearings. Drama as a distortion of reality can emotionally consume and distract a clinician from competent clinical practice. The irony of it all is that some doyens and doyennes have polished approaches of instigating drama to attack and sabotage new employees considered to be threats. They have been able to control others with such drama. The drama can be a vehicle for delivering abusive and vicious attacks where naïve individuals lacking insight into drama get professionally and emotionally injured. A clinician wishing to engage in the game of dealing with toxic and dysfunctional situations will need to present with integrity and character using the motivations of principles and ethics.

Every organization has its dysfunction or toxicity, and its discovery is part of a decision-making process by the clinician as to whether a problem exists that requires a response. Furthermore, even in the face of honorable intentions and solid ethical values, many hostile work situations present as immutable to change due to an entrenched status quo of dysfunctional individuals exercising rigid control. A clinician may be faced with the complex choice of determining whether the toxicity and hostility of the workplace can be tolerated and kept from interfering with the delivery of competent clinical service.

In the end, a clinician becomes a clinician to help people and not to waste time and energy responding to the distraction of workplace drama. However, it is a reality, and hopefully more clinicians can cooperatively engage in intentional ways of managing drama in clinical settings such as PHP/IOP settings and making them fulfilling places in which to work.

REFERENCES

Berne, E. (2004). *Games people play*. New York, NY: Ballantine Books. (Original work published 1964)

Brendtro, L. K., & Mitchell, M. (1983). The organizational ethos: From tension to teamwork. In L. K. Brendtro & A. E. Ness (Eds.), *Re-educating trouble youth: Environments for teaching and treatment*. Hawthorne, NY: Aldine.

Centers for Disease Control and Prevention. (2010). *Selected findings for the healthcare sector by occupation from the 2010 National Health Interview Survey—Occupational Health Supplement (NHIS-OHS)*. Retrieved from http://www.cdc.gov/niosh/topics/nhis/pdfs/HealthcareOccupationProfile.pdf

Kübler-Ross, E. (1969). *On death and dying*. New York, NY: Scribner.

CHAPTER SEVENTEEN

CONCLUDING THOUGHTS

*T*here has been no other significant, new book on partial hospitaliza-tion program (PHP)/intensive outpatient program (IOP) practice for over three decades. This is unfortunate, given the evolution both in how the average PHP/IOP is conducted and in how this level of care is being adapted for use with an increasing variety of patient cohorts. This book is an effort to fill the need for relevant, general guidance and direction on providing clinical services to multiple PHP/IOP cohorts that reflects the current state of affairs.

In the effort to generalize, a pattern was followed in each chapter. First, analysis was conducted on a significant practice aspect in terms of its typical challenges. Second, an adaptation of Norton Long's (1958) *ecology of games* theory was conceptualized for each aspect as a set of suggested practice strategies needed to address the challenges. The detail and complexity of the strategies varied, based on the aspect of practice. Markers of practice success were identified where applicable. The intent of using this pattern was to conceptualize a theoretical order for both appraisal and action in an otherwise complex and intense clin-ical practice setting.

Hopefully, the reader can utilize the conceptualizations of order to appreciate clinical and relational situations in both cross-sectional and longitudinal dimensions. Understanding and managing some clinical sit-uations requires cross-sectional analysis of the current phenomena. The management of other clinical situations requires analyzing sequences of events. Some complex clinical situations will require both analyses in order to choose effective interventions or address problems.

Besides the theoretical conception of order, this book sought to be different in that it empathizes with the clinician. The complexity and intensity prevalent in the various aspects of the PHP/IOP setting can be daunting at times. Throughout the book, an effort was made to illu-minate this emotional intensity and suggest cues on how a clinician can respond with professional composure and perspective so as to manage the emotionally challenging PHP/IOP situations and crises. The intent of this empathetic thread was to guide newer clinicians onto a meaningful and satisfying trajectory of professional development and to enrich experienced clinicians.

REFERENCE

Long, N. (1958). The local community as an ecology of games. *American Journal of Sociology, 64*, 251–261.

EXAMPLE OF AN INITIAL TREATMENT PLANNING SURVEY

NAME: _____   DATE: _____

How are you feeling today? (PLEASE CIRCLE your choices) sad, happy, mad, numb, anxious, worried, confused, overwhelmed, relieved, frightened, tired, depressed, or write other: _____
_____

In your own words, what happened that you needed to come to us for our services? _____
_____
_____
_____

In your own words, what do you need from our services?
_____
_____
_____
_____

If you just came from the inpatient unit (upstairs), do you feel that you made progress? If so, how? _____
_____

In your own words, what do you feel you need to change or accomplish?
_____
_____
_____
_____

Circle your answer: 0 = none; 10 = the WORST

Depression Score: 0 1 2 3 4 5 6 7 8 9 10

Anxiety Score: 0 1 2 3 4 5 6 7 8 9 10

Have you had or are you having any hallucinations?
(Hearing or seeing things.)   YES ___   NO ___

Do you feel paranoid, as if someone is watching you?
                         YES ___   NO ___   AT TIMES: ___

Circle your answer: 0 = none; 10 = the WORST

Paranoia Score: 0 1 2 3 4 5 6 7 8 9 10

Are you having any thoughts of wanting to hurt others or kill someone?
                                          YES ___   NO ___

Are you having any thoughts of wanting to kill yourself/hurt yourself or
wanting to die?   YES ___   NO ___

Are you taking your medications as the doctor prescribed them?
                                          YES ___   NO ___
Are you feeling any benefit from your medication?/Is it helping?
                                          YES___   NO ___
Are you having any side effects from the medication? YES ___   NO ___
Have you had any changes in your medication?   YES ___   NO ___
If yes, what are the changes? _____

Did you use any alcohol in the past week? YES ___ NO ___ If yes, what
kind?
_____

Did you use any street or unprescribed drugs in the past week?
YES ___ NO ___ What? _____

Do you normally drink alcohol or use recreational substances?
                                   YES _____ NO _____

Are you craving alcohol or recreational substances?

YES _____ NO _____

Circle your answer: 0 = none; 10 = the WORST

Craving Score: 0 1 2 3 4 5 6 7 8 9 10

Did you use any OVER-THE-COUNTER drugs in the past week?
YES _____ NO _____ What? _____

How is your concentration?   GOOD   FAIR   POOR

How is your appetite?   GOOD   FAIR   POOR
_____ Meals _____ Snacks yesterday

How many hours of sleep did you get last night? _____
Indicate whether it was good, fair, or restless.

Family Questions

Who lives in your home? _____
How are things in your home? _____
Is your family in town or out of town? _____
Are things good with your family or do you avoid them?_____
_____

Does anyone in your family have a history of mental health problems?
YES _____ NO _____ WHO? _____

Does anyone in your family have a history of drug/alcohol problems?
YES _____ NO _____ WHO? _____

Any problems with family that are really bothering you? If so, what?
_____

Personal History

Have you ever been the victim or survivor of any trauma or abuse? If so,
what?_____
_____

Do you have legal issues or court dates?

_____

Do you have financial stresses or problems? If yes, what?

_____

Did you go to any 12-step meetings (AA, NA, OA, Al-Anon) in the past week?   YES ___ NO ___

Do you have any new employer problems or problems getting work? YES ___ NO ___ If yes, what are the problems? _____

_____

Have you met with Vocational Rehabilitation? YES ___ NO ___. Do you want to? YES ___ NO ___. If you have already, what is your progress?

_____

_____

Are you trying to get long-term or short-term disability? YES ___ NO ___ If yes, what is your progress?

Do you have an outside psychiatrist appointment? YES ___ NO ___ If yes, when is it?

_____

Do you have an outside counselor/therapist? YES ___ NO ___ If yes, when is your next appointment?

_____

Would you like to get an outside therapist or psychiatrist, if you do not have one? YES ___ NO ___

How much longer do you see yourself in this program?

_____

Any other comments that can help us give you effective and excellent care?

_____

_____

EXAMPLE OF A CONCURRENT TREATMENT PLANNING SURVEY

(PLEASE COMPLETE ALL PAGES)

NAME: _____   DATE: _____

How are you feeling today? (PLEASE CIRCLE your choices) sad, happy, mad, numb, anxious, worried, confused, overwhelmed, relieved, frightened, tired, depressed, or other: _____
_____

Do you remember what the treatment plan goals were last week?
                                        YES _____   NO _____

In your own words, how do you see your progress in this program in the past week? Did you have any accomplishments?
_____
_____
_____
_____

In your own words, what do you feel you need to work more on <u>or to accomplish</u>?
_____
_____

Did you do anything else for your recovery in the past week that you felt helped you move along?
_____
_____
_____

What did not work for you in the last week that you tried to help you recover?

_____

_____

Circle your answer: 0 = none; 10 = the WORST

Depression Score: 0 1 2 3 4 5 6 7 8 9 10

Anxiety Score: 0 1 2 3 4 5 6 7 8 9 10

Have you had or are you having any hallucinations?   YES ___ NO ___

Do you feel paranoid, as if someone is watching you?
                              YES ___ NO ___ AT TIMES: __

Circle your answer: 0 = none; 10 = the WORST

Paranoia Score: 0 1 2 3 4 5 6 7 8 9 10

Have you had any thoughts of wanting to hurt others or kill someone?
                              YES ___ NO ___

Any thoughts of wanting to kill yourself/hurt yourself or wanting
to die?   YES ___ NO ___

Are you taking your medications as the doctor prescribed them?
                              YES ___ NO ___

Are you feeling any benefit from your medication?/Are they helping?
                              YES ___ NO ___

Are you having any side effects from the medication?   YES ___ NO ___

Have you had any changes in your medication?   YES ___ NO ___

If yes, what are the changes? _____

_____

Did you use any alcohol in the past week? YES _____ NO _____
If yes, what kind? _____

Did you use any street or unprescribed drugs in the past week?
                    YES _____ NO _____ What? _____

Circle your answer: 0 = none; 10 = the WORST

Craving Score: 0 1 2 3 4 5 6 7 8 9 10

Did you use any OVER-THE-COUNTER drugs in the past week?
                    YES _____ NO _____ What? _____

How is your concentration?   GOOD   FAIR   POOR

How is your appetite?   GOOD   FAIR   POOR
                               ____ Meals ____ Snacks yesterday
How many hours of sleep did you get last night? _____
                    Indicate whether it was good, fair, or restless.

Do you have **any new** legal issues or court dates?
_____

Do you have **any new** financial stresses or problems? If yes, what?
_____

Do you have any new employer problems or problems getting work?
YES ___ NO ___ If yes, what are the problems? _____
_____

Have you met with Vocational Rehabilitation?   YES ___ NO ___
Do you want to? YES ___ NO ___ If you have already, what is your
progress?
_____

Are you trying to get long-term or short-term disability? YES ___ NO ___
If yes, what is your progress? _____
_____

Do you have an outside psychiatrist appointment? YES ___ NO ___
If yes, when is it? _____
_____

Do you have an outside counselor/therapist? YES ___ NO ___ If yes,
when is your next appointment? _____
_____

Would you like to get an outside therapist or psychiatrist, if you do not
have one?   YES ___ NO ___

Have you gone to any support groups this week such as Al-Anon or AA?
                                                              YES ___ NO ___

How much longer do you see yourself in this program?
_____

Any other comments that can help us give you effective and excellent
care?
_____
_____
_____
_____

EXAMPLE OF A FAX
TRANSMISSION LEAD SHEET

Fax Transmission Lead Sheet

Smith Hospital PHP/IOP

Phone: 502-555-3019 Fax: 502-555-3128

To: Psychiatric Associates   Phone: 502-555-1234, Fax: 502-555-1235

From **[Clinician Name Here]**

Dr Beell ordered follow-up for the following patient with himself:

Mary Smith (DOB 01-19-1967)
Good Health Insurance Policy: P1834897, GRP 30183
Phone number: 502-555-2969
Address:
8909 Indianapolis Rd
Louisville, KY 40272

Please call me at 502-555-3048 with the appointment time and I will notify the patient.

> This is an example of a recommended, one-page fax template for making aftercare appointments with a psychiatric practice. It is a one-page file saved on a hard drive that can be edited each and every time for a new patient.

EXAMPLES OF A DAILY ASSESSMENT FORM

EXAMPLE #1

NAME: _____   DATE:_____

1. What are your feelings today? (PLEASE CIRCLE) sad, happy, numb, confused, overwhelmed, relieved, frightened, or write other: _____
   _____
   _____

2. Please circle a number for both (0 = coping; 10 = very poor coping).

   Depression: 0 1 2 3 4 5 6 7 8 9 10
   Anxiety: 0 1 2 3 4 5 6 7 8 9 10

3. Do you have any thoughts of suicide or wanting to hurt yourself?
   YES or NO (please circle)
4. Do you have any thoughts of wanting to hurt or kill another person?
   YES or NO (please circle)
5. Are your medications helping? YES or NO?
6. Are you taking the medications as the doctor prescribed them?
   YES or NO?
7. Are there any changes in your medication? YES or NO? If yes, what?
   _____
8. How many hours of sleep did you get last night? _____ Was the sleep good, fair, poor? Did you wake up early?
9. How was your appetite yesterday? Good? Fair? Poor?
10. How is your concentration? Good? Fair? Poor?

11. Circle your concerns today: medications, anxiety, depression, problem solving, stress, communication, relationships
12. Do you have a goal for therapy today? What is it? _____

_____

EXAMPLE #2

NAME: _____   DATE: _____

1. How are you feeling today? (Please circle your choices) sad, happy, angry, depressed, numb, anxious, confused, overwhelmed, relieved, frightened, or other:_____

_____

2. Please circle a rating for each of the following: (0 = coping; 10 = not coping at all)

   Depression: 0 1 2 3 4 5 6 7 8 9 10
   Anxiety: 0 1 2 3 4 5 6 7 8 9 10

3. Are you having any of the following? (Circle your answer):
   • Any thoughts of wanting to hurt yourself?   YES/NO
   • Any thoughts of wanting to commit suicide?   YES/NO
   • Any thoughts of wanting to die?   YES/NO
   • Any thoughts of wanting to not wake up?   YES/NO
   • Any thoughts of wanting to wanting to kill, hurt, or injure another person?   YES/NO

4. Are your medications helping? _____
5. Are you taking your medications as prescribed? _____
6. Any changes in medications? _____ If so, what are they?

_____

7. Last night I slept _____ hours and slept (circle all that apply) poor, restless, early awakening, good, slept too much, or other

   _____

8. My appetite is (circle one) poor, fair, good, eat too much, or other; I ate ___ meals and ___ snacks.
9. My concentration is (circle one) poor, fair, good, or other

   _____

10. My concerns include (circle all that apply):
   Medications   Anxiety   Depression   Problem solving
   Stress   Relationships   Communication
11. My goals in therapy today are: _____

_____

EXAMPLE #3

Your Name: _____   Today's Date: _____

Please check your feeling(s)

o sad   o confused
o happy   o overwhelmed
o angry   o relieved
o depressed   o frightened
o numb   o other _____
o anxious/nervous
                               _____

Are you having any of the following?

Thoughts of wanting to hurt yourself?   o YES   o NO
Thoughts of wanting to commit suicide?   o YES   o NO
Thoughts of wanting to die?   o YES   o NO
Thoughts of wanting to not wake up?   o YES   o NO
Thoughts of wanting to kill, hurt, or
injure another person?   o YES   o NO

Please circle your depression score

0	1–2	3–4	5–6	7–8	9–10
Not depressed	Down/ mild depression	Sad/ moderate depression	Blue/severe depression	Unhappy/ very severe depression	Hopeless/ suicidal/ worst possible depression

Please circle your anxiety score

0	1–2	3–4	5–6	7–8	9–10
Not anxious	Concerned/ tense/mild anxiety	Worried/ moderate anxiety	Nervous/ jumpy/severe anxiety	Fearful/ very severe anxiety	Panic attacks/ worst possible anxiety

How are the following?

Appetite	o Good	o Fair	o Poor
Sleep	o Good	o Fair	o Poor
Concentration	o Good	o Fair	o Poor

What are your concerns today?

o Medications	o Stress	o Something else_____
o Anxiety	o Relationships	_____
o Depression	o Communication	_____
o Problem solving	o Work	

Index

Lightning Source UK Ltd.
Milton Keynes UK
UKOW06f0345131115

262569UK00001B/121/P